T0310645

Learning and Behaviour
in Medicine

Learning and Behaviour in Medicine
A Voyage Around CME and CPD

Robin Stevenson
Editor-in-Chief, *Journal of European CME*
Honorary Professor of Medicine
Glasgow University, UK

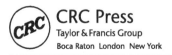

CRC Press
Taylor & Francis Group
Boca Raton London New York

CRC Press is an imprint of the
Taylor & Francis Group, an **informa** business

First edition published 2022
by CRC Press
6000 Broken Sound Parkway NW, Suite 300, Boca Raton, FL 33487-2742

and by CRC Press
4 Park Square, Milton Park, Abingdon, Oxon, OX14 4RN

CRC Press is an imprint of Taylor & Francis Group, LLC

Trademark notice: Product or corporate names may be trademarks or registered trademarks and are used only for identification and explanation without intent to infringe.

ISBN: 9781032218410 (hbk)
ISBN: 9781032218458 (pbk)
ISBN: 9781003270287 (ebk)

DOI: 10.1201/9781003270287

Typeset in Times
by codeMantra

Contents

Prologue

To read this book is to embark on a voyage around CME and CPD with nine ports-of-call each represented by a chapter. The readership comprises groups of *passengers* all curious to learn more about the ports-of-call and hopeful of being enlightened and enriched by the experience.

Who should accompany the author on his voyage? The CME and CPD cognoscenti will have travelled this way before and may find the voyage too short, with not enough time to spend exploring all the fascinating places on the way. They may however be interested to compare the perspective of a clinician with that of an educationalist.

The voyage may be better suited to health professionals who have only a passing acquaintance with CME and CPD, people who sail in and out of the CME/CPD world without ever quite understanding what it is all about. Among them, many of the physicians* will have collected their credits completely unaware of the educational hinterland of CME or how it is different from their undergraduate and graduate education. It is one of the aims of this voyage to show learners how to approach CME and CPD in such a way that their clinical practice will be improved by their participation in this learning experience.

Another group of passengers who might benefit from the voyage are people who find themselves involved in the provision of CME, not as full-time professionals but as amateurs. Physicians, by virtue of membership of specialist societies, are often parachuted into education committees which have to organise CME for the members. If they are lucky, staff members may show them the ropes, but not all staff are familiar with CME. The amateurs first have to realise that there is more to CME than they thought and that they should learn the rules about how to plan and deliver it and how to assess its effectiveness. Perhaps, sailing on this short voyage will help them to do that.

There is a particular reason to welcome CME providers from Europe. These include not only specialist society providers but also professional providers. On the voyage they will discover that the United States and Canada

---

* In this book, the term "physician" is used generically to indicate any medically qualified healthcare professional and therefore includes surgeons, GPs, psychiatrists, etc.

have led the way in developing CME and CPD and that Europe has lagged behind. They may think that they are disadvantaged in comparison with their North American counterparts, especially in relation to the regulations governing the provision of CME. If so, they may feel moved to make their concerns known to the European national regulatory authorities.

It follows therefore that those who supervise and regulate the provision and usage of CME and those who accredit its quality might also benefit from being on the voyage. Passengers in these groups from different countries and continents could compare their practices. The accreditors divided by the Atlantic Ocean may be able to explore the possibility of reaching a consensus on how best to assure the quality of education available to healthcare professionals.

The last group to be invited on the voyage are academics interested in all aspects of education, including undergraduate medical education. They will be surprised to discover that almost all of the important research into CME and CPD has been carried out in academic institutions in North America. They will ask themselves why Europe and the rest of the world have contributed so little. The author hopes that their dialogue with the CME community during the voyage will provide the answer to their question and perhaps point to a solution to the problem.

Acknowledgements

The author is grateful to Murray Kopelow, Cara Macfarlane, Graham McMahon, Lewis Miller, Don Moore and Eugene Pozniak for sharing their knowledge with him and for their helpful suggestions.

Abbreviations

AAFP	American Association of Family Physicians
ACCME	Accreditation Council for CME
CME	Continuing Medical Education
CPD	Continuing Professional Development
CT	Computerised tomography
CTC	Commitment to change
DE	Distractor efficiency
DI	Discrimination Index
DIF I	Difficulty Index
EEA	European Economic Area
EACCME	European Accreditation Council for CME
ERS	European Respiratory Society
EU	European Union
GP	General practitioner
IPCE	Interprofessional CME
IPE	Interprofessional education (formal)
IPL	Interprofessional learning (informal)
IPTM	Interprofessional team meeting
ITU	Intensive therapy unit
MCQ	Multiple-choice questions
MDTM	Multi-disciplinary team meeting
MOC	Maintenance of Certification
MRI	Magnetic resonance imaging
MSF	Multi-source feedback
NAA	National Accreditation Authority
NFD	Non-functional distractor
NHS	National Health Service
OR	Odds ratio
PI CME	Performance Improvement CME
PPG	Professional practice gap
Q&A	Question and answer
QI	Quality improvement
RCT	Randomised control trial
RD	Risk difference

RR	Relative risk
SD	Standard deviation
UEMS	Union of European Medical Specialists
UK	United Kingdom
US	United States

The Beginning of CME and Its Relationship to CPD

1

Physicians have always gathered together to listen to their senior colleagues hoping to improve their own clinical practice, learn of new developments and to meet physicians from other places and other specialties. From such seeds has grown a new discipline.

In the 1930s, Continuing Medical Education (CME) entered physicians' lexicon and was accepted as being limited to that learning relevant to their professional behaviour. "CME is a systematic attempt to facilitate change in doctors' practice" was suggested as a succinct definition by Fox [1]. Initially, it followed the style of existing education in medical schools by being mainly didactic, prescriptive and non-interactive. By the 1980s, studies had been published showing that this form of CME had little effect on physicians' behaviour or patient health [2]. The response to this in North America was to experiment with CME design and delivery in an attempt to improve its effectiveness.

At the same time in the United Kingdom (UK), the whole concept of traditional, didactic CME was challenged as being too restrictive and only concerned with the competencies of clinical practice. Physicians were thought to need skills encompassing not just clinical practice but also personal appraisals, coping strategies, management, inter-professional relationships, clinical audit, information technology and communication abilities. This all-embracing prospectus was to be called Continuing Professional Development (CPD), of

DOI: 10.1201/9781003270287-1

which CME was to be an important part [3]. Davis and colleagues in 2003 went further and suggested using the term CPD exclusively and discarding CME because of its connotation with lectures in darkened rooms [4].

While the terminology surrounding CME was being discussed in high places, the studies on how best to deliver it were bearing fruit. Eight systematic reviews were published (seven in the first decade of the new century) which showed that when CME was delivered in accordance with specific educational criteria, both physician performance and patient health improved [5].

Although early bicycles were replaced by bicycles with gears without the need to invent a new name for bicycles, the CME detractors' enthusiasm for the name change to CPD was undiminished. Some countries such as the UK and Canada have replaced CME entirely by CPD and some others in Europe have used the hybrid CME/CPD. Regardless of which name is used, there seems to be no discernible difference in practice between countries that refer to CME, CME/CPD or CPD alone. Equivalent credits are awarded to participants irrespective of the name of the system. CPD apologists therefore argue that nothing has been lost in consigning CME to the rubbish bin, a view endorsed by people who think *medical* is elitist and non-inclusive.

The lumpers seem to have won the day, but the splitters should have their say. They point out that CME is specific for healthcare workers involved in *medicine* and that *education* can be measured both in content and effect and appropriate recognition granted. On the other hand, CPD is applicable to any profession, and *development* just means change for better or for worse. It is doubtful whether development can be delivered by a third party. Credits can be awarded to learners shown to have been *educated*, but how can participants in so-called CPD be shown to have *developed* and thereby qualify for credits?

Splitters see obvious value in the concept of CPD, but say that it is more complex and less easily quantified than CME. It implies behavioural change that arises in an individual physician in response to changes in the working environment peculiar to that physician. As such, it can only be measured by personal appraisal, peer review or multi-source feedback. It may be influenced by CME but can occur independently of it. On occasions both may be involved. For example, a hospital CME department may be investigating a presumed practice gap in a diabetic clinic where performance is sub-optimal. It discovers the cause when the clinic manager is found to be a misogynistic bully. There is no obvious educative solution to this problem. If the manager was medical, they could be offered remedial CME, but without much hope of success [6]. The medical staff must work out how to deal with the manager and if they succeed, their success can be attributed to that part of their CPD that deals with people skills.

Unlike CME, there is no evidence that planned CPD affects physicians' performance, and therefore to reward such CPD activities with credit points may be questionable. In a sense, CME helps physicians to treat their patients, whereas with CPD, the physicians themselves are the patients. Just because

CPD cannot be formally learnt, does not mean that it is not important and should not be evaluated. Maintenance of Certification and revalidation are wholly dependent on CPD assessment. This includes not only the contribution of CME but also the effects of age, cognitive decline, interpersonal difficulties, substance abuse and communication problems, all of which are relevant to fitness to practise. Advancing age is one of the main determinants of clinical performance [7], and behavioural assessment is at least as important as CME in determining whether physicians should be recertified or revalidated.

The splitters argue that the healthcare professions would benefit from making a clear distinction between CME and CPD, which are still relative newcomers to the medical establishment and yet to be accepted by many practising physicians as important and necessary to their profession. Their cause is not helped when both terms are used loosely. The recently founded *International Academy for CPD Accreditation* states that CME is often used interchangeably with CPD. It then adds to the confusion by saying that "Continuing professional development is a scholarly pursuit ... and CME is the academy in which it occurs". Despite the International Academy's avowed alignment with CPD accreditation, five of the six domains in its recent *Standards for Substantive Equivalency* are devoted to education [8]. The lack of precise definition detracts from the credibility of a concept.

CME was mainly nurtured in the United States (US), but the name is falling out of favour in some organisations because *medicine* does not sit well with the current advocacy of interprofessional education. The survival of CME in America may have been helped by its being embedded in ACCME, the Accreditation Council for CME, which is the world's oldest and best known accreditation agency. So although the establishment would like to change to CE (Continuing Education) or CPD, the old name is still often heard in a country that continues to use the imperial measures of inches, feet and yards. The one-time imperial power has of course embraced metric measurement along with CPD. Apart from the UK, Europe seems comfortable with both the decimal system of measurement and with CME as a descriptor. In the future, perhaps the flags of both CME and CPD will fly in the first port-of-call in our voyage.

REFERENCES

1. Fox RD, Bennett NL. Learning and change: implications for continuing medical education. *BMJ* 1998;316:466–468.
2. Lloyd JS, Abrahamson S. Effectiveness of continuing medical education: a review of the evidence. *Evaluation & the Health Professions* 1979;2:251–280.

3. Atlay RD, Wentz DK. CME or CPD? *Postgraduate Medical Journal* 1996;72(suppl):S613.
4. Davis D, Barnes BE, Fox RD. *The Continuing Professional Development of Physicians: From Research to Practice.* American Medical Association (AMA), Chicago; 2003.
5. Cervero RM, Gaines JK. The impact of CME on physician performance and patient health outcomes: an updated synthesis of systematic reviews. *Journal of Continuing Education in the Health Professions* 2015;35(2):131–138.
6. Hanna E, Premi J, Turnbull J. Results of remedial continuing medical education in dyscompetent physicians. *Academic Medicine* 2000;75(2):174–176.
7. Choudhry NK, Fletcher RH, Soumerai SB. Systematic review: the relationship between clinical experience and the quality of health care. *Annals of Internal Medicine* 2005;142(4):260–736.
8. International Academy for Accreditation in CPD. https://academy4cpd-accreditation.org/about-us/

Culture of Learning 2

The CME community has an interest in the reasons why healthcare people learn. They learn to obtain professional qualifications and learn again in subsequent training to become competent in their specialties. Outside medicine, they learn to play games, engage in sport, play musical instruments, speak foreign languages and bring up children. Sometimes they just learn to satisfy their curiosity. The motive for this kind of learning is entirely selfish. The reward for learning is the happiness experienced by the learner and its motivation is multi-faceted with both intrinsic and extrinsic components [1].

Healthcare organisations must encourage their members to learn so that they can contribute better to the success of the organisation. Here the motive of the learners is unselfish in that it does not lead directly to increased prosperity or happiness. Successful organisations bring their culture to bear on their members to encourage them to learn. Organisational culture is an expression of the values and assumptions of the people working in the organisation often built up over many years. These values may be passed down, often unconsciously, from one generation to the next [2]. Therefore, when leading figures in the organisation display a firm commitment to teaching and learning, these values become embedded in the fabric of the organisation and younger members unconsciously absorb them. This motivation may be described as intrinsic in contrast to extrinsic where learning would be rewarded by promotion or bonus payments [3]. Organisations increasingly believe that they are better served by intrinsic than by extrinsic motivation. Intrinsically motivated cadets at West Point in the US were more likely to be promoted and stay in the army than cadets who were extrinsically motivated [4].

In the healthcare world, recent rearrangements of professional relationships have made necessary a radical reappraisal of its cultural values and assumptions. In previous times, hierarchical structures in all healthcare professions strengthened the cultural assumptions of teaching and learning. Senior physicians regularly taught medical students at the bedside. They usually attended clinical meetings where juniors presented cases for discussion. The much-maligned entourages on ward rounds allowed juniors to learn from seniors and vice versa. Nevertheless, in the present day, traditional medical hierarchy is rightly criticised for having fostered a deferential culture and being the enemy of team-working. This fundamental attitudinal change in modern healthcare has meant that status now relates more to competence and expertise than to seniority. The downside is that physicians, so preoccupied with their own performance, tend to be forgetful of their profession's time-honoured responsibility for learning and teaching.

The supplanting by meritocracy of hierarchy based on seniority left a leadership vacuum, which has been filled by insurance companies, a managerial class or a politicised bureaucracy. Of these, the last is the least successful, exemplified by the UK where almost 8,000 doctors were recently surveyed. Many reported a culture of fear and blame and about half of them said they did not have the time to learn and develop professionally in their role. The report called for a fundamental shift in culture to a genuinely supportive learning environment [5]. It is not surprising that the largest National Health Service (NHS)-governing body, NHS England, employing 6,500 people, has not a single NHS clinician among its 16 directors [6]. Physicians working in such healthcare organisations are careless of their duty to teach and to learn, feel a loss of status and often seek early retirement [7,8].

In countries where fully socialised healthcare has not been adopted, insurance companies and hospital managers have picked up the mantle of leadership laid down by the old hierarchy. Their hospitals have to survive in a competitive environment where good performance is financially rewarded. Such institutions are therefore motivated to invest in their people and to encourage CME knowing its potential effect on clinical performance [9]. Leadership of this kind promotes a culture of learning, which obliges physicians to teach as well as to learn. They feel valued in this environment and take pride in their profession and in its collegiate and academic institutions. They tend not to take early retirement.

To be part of a learning culture is a privilege which is not only rewarding in itself but also conducive to improved clinical practice. National governments know that health professionals must engage in continuing education, but instead of fostering a culture where people want to learn, they impose mandatory criteria in an attempt to ensure adequate CME. The various systems in individual countries are basically similar [10] and need not be described here, but it is doubtful whether a regulatory approach will encourage a learning culture as effectively as intelligent management systems operating at local levels.

It is increasingly recognised by good management that formal external CME has less effect on clinical practice than workplace CME. This can be organised and promoted by hospital CME departments, common in the US, but rare in Europe. In the US in 2019, almost 50,000 CME activities were delivered within the hospital/healthcare system, which exceeded the number of activities delivered by physician membership organisations, education companies or medical schools [11]. Team-working spontaneously creates multi-disciplinary and interprofessional team meetings, which have major educational potential. Point-of-care CME using mobile devices has become a fact of medical life. Teaching at the bedside and in the clinic contributes to the hospital's reputation. Therefore, despite this revolution, in which the *Ancien Régime* of hierarchy and privilege has been supplanted by meritocracy and team-working, there is good reason to believe that a culture of learning will survive and prosper provided that political interference is resisted. And so we can sail away from our second port-of-call with guarded optimism.

REFERENCES

1. Reiss S. Intrinsic and extrinsic motivation. *Teaching of Psychology* 2012;39(2):152–156. doi:10.1177/0098628312437704
2. Schein EH. Organizational culture. *American Psychologist* 1990;45(2):109–119.
3. Legault L. Intrinsic and extrinsic motivation. In: Zeigler-Hill V., Shackelford T. (eds) *Encyclopedia of Personality and Individual Differences*. Springer, Cham; 2016. https://doi.org/10.1007/978-3-319-28099-8_1139-1
4. Intrinsic motivation West Point. https://www.fastcompany.com/3047370/the-only-type-of-motivation-that-leads-to-success
5. Survey of UK doctors highlights blame culture within the NHS. https://www.bmj.com/content/362/bmj.k4001.full
6. NHS England. Board Members 2021 https://www.england.nhs.uk/about/board/nhs-england-board/members
7. Stevenson RD, Moore DE. A culture of learning for the NHS. *Journal of European CME* 2019;8:1. doi:10.1080/21614083.2019.1613862
8. Stevenson RD. Why the NHS needs a culture shift from blame and fear to learning. https://theconversation.com/why-the-nhs-needs-a-culture-shift-from-blame-and-fear-to-learning–118707
9. Cervero RM, Gaines JK. The impact of CME on physician performance and patient health outcomes: an updated synthesis of systematic reviews. *Journal of Continuing Education in the Health Professions* 2015;35(2):131–138.
10. IOM (Institute of Medicine). *Redesigning Continuing Education in the Health Professions. Appendix C, International Comparison of Continuing Education and Continuing Professional Development*. The National Academies Press, Washington, DC; 2010. https://www.ncbi.nlm.nih.gov/books/NBK219811/?report=reader
11. Accreditation Council for Continuing Medical Education. ACCME Data Report: Steady Growth in Accredited Continuing Medical Education – 2019. 2020. www.accme.org/2019datareport. https://www.accme.org/sites/default/files/2020-07/872_2020%2007%2028_2019_Data_Report.pdf

Professional Practice Gap and the CME Community

3

Some medical educators still regard CME as simply an extension of undergraduate education and graduate training, based on a rolling curriculum covering all aspects of the relevant medical specialty and delivered mainly by didactic teaching. They should be aware of the impressive body of evidence, which has shown that this approach improves neither physicians' performance nor patient health [1–5].

Having appreciated this disturbing discovery, the CME community embarked on a huge effort to find out how to plan and deliver CME, so that physicians could be persuaded to change their behaviour to improve patient care. In 1983, Robert Fox started the ball rolling by introducing the concept of *discrepancy* as the distance between *what is* and *what should be* [6]. Discrepancies in patient health may happen for many reasons, including societal problems of poverty, bad living conditions and despair, and for these, the CME planner has little to offer. But when analysis of the discrepancy or gap does suggest inadequate physician performance, the planner must ask whether this is due to deficiency of physician knowledge, skills or attitude, or other factors affecting performance such as system failure. If the analysis confirms the culprit to be physician behaviour, the planner must design CME appropriate for the particular problem that has been demonstrated.

In other words, when the discrepancy or gap is related to physician performance, it defines the medical educational need and the analytic process leading to this conclusion is described as *needs assessment*. In this book, the term *gap analysis* will be preferred to *needs assessment* because it defines the process more expressively. This approach is in accord with the principles of adult learning published a decade earlier by Knowles [7]. The American educator's assumptions of adult learning included *orientation to learning* in which learning is problem-centred instead of subject-centred in direct contrast to children's learning. In the language of the educational psychologist, CME is to undergraduate education what andragogy is to pedagogy, and the learner must be actively rather than passively involved as described by Benjamin Franklin:

> *Tell me and I forget, teach me and I may remember, involve me and I learn.*

Converted to this new philosophy, CME planners and providers discarded the term *discrepancy* and replaced it with *professional practice gap* (PPG) and gave it pride of place in their educational resources. In addition, they favoured interactive rather than passive learning and distanced themselves from didactic lectures. They experimented with multi-media delivery of CME, formative assessment with feedback, repetition and reinforcement. They presented physicians with the evidence suggesting the presence of a PPG with the implication that it was caused by their inadequate performance. Receipt of such unwelcome information made the physicians feel uncomfortable, a state of mind described as *cognitive dissonance* [8]. The purpose of inducing this mental discomfort was to create a *teachable moment* when it was hoped that physicians would become predisposed to learn from a CME intervention [9]. Gradually, their efforts were rewarded by evidence that their new approach was working with increasing numbers of studies showing definite effects on physician knowledge and performance with lesser effects on patient health [10–14].

More recently, a comprehensive and detailed analysis was carried out on eight systematic reviews of CME effectiveness published after 2003. Five of them found that both physician performance and patient health were affected by CME and that the effect on performance was greater than the effect on patient health. All eight reviews showed that the effect was increased when the CME is "more interactive, uses more methods, involves multiple exposures, is longer and is focused on outcomes that are considered important by physicians" [15].

This was a monumental research effort, almost entirely carried out in Canada and the US and comprising many hundreds of studies. But the message has not travelled well, both in North America and across the Atlantic. CME professionals either failed to engage with the medical establishment or did engage with it but failed to persuade sceptical clinicians of the validity and relevance of their message. They have not been offered membership of the exclusive establishment clubs, the most powerful and influential of which are the national and international specialist societies. Many of these societies have taken the Olympian view that they needed no lessons in the planning and delivery of education to their members. This is doubly disappointing since the societies are major providers of CME. Until the pandemic, they still organised huge annual congresses dominated by didactic lectures, with little attempt to seek out PPGs or otherwise adopt the tenets of modern CME so painstakingly elaborated.

Many CME professionals have had experiences confirming that the medical establishment has not yet embraced modern CME practice. The author was recently involved in a series of teleconferences with representatives of the European specialist societies. It was surprising to discover how many of them had never heard of Moore's Outcomes Pyramid (Chapter 5) or of a PPG. Consequently, their ideas about CME were rooted in their undergraduate experience of curricular education. They were almost universally resistant to the proposition that CME should be a reparative process occasioned by the discovery of a discrepancy or practice gap in clinical practice. The concept of adult education being problem-centred was foreign to them.

THE CME COMMUNITY

This period of intense activity could be said to mark the coming of age of the CME community, which was largely a North American development and was based in the education departments of university medical schools in the US and Canada. Membership initially comprised a mixture of physicians and educationalists and later welcomed academic nurses, pharmacists and commercial CME providers.

It had already created the structures characteristic of a healthcare specialty. Its largest organisation is the *Alliance for Continuing Education in the Health Professions* originally founded in the US as the *Alliance for Continuing Medical Education* in 1975 on the instigation of Lewis Miller. *Möbius* was the first journal dedicated to CME, published in 1981, and changed its name in 1988 to the *Journal of Continuing Education in the Health Professions*.

The *Global Alliance for Medical Education* (GAME) was established in 1995, again by Lewis Miller, as a CME discussion forum mainly for commercial providers. A not-for-profit, educational organisation, the *European CME Forum* (ECF) was set up in the UK by Eugene Pozniak in 2008 with annual meetings in European cities. The ECF introduced the *Journal of European CME* in 2012. The *Good CME Practice Group* was created in 2009, again by Eugene Pozniak, with membership restricted to independent CME providers.

The most important and pressing challenge facing the leadership of the CME community is its failure to integrate fully with the body politic of the healthcare professions. Many of the leaders in North American CME have been educationalists who speak and write in their own language, which is often incomprehensible to clinicians. There is a subtle difference between self-efficacy and self-confidence, which educationalists appreciate but which would be lost on clinicians. In Europe, educationalists specialising in CME are rare, because CME has not been accepted as an academic discipline by medical schools and universities and has not developed a tradition of scholarly research.

The European CME contingent, perhaps emboldened by the success of the ECF, has been making overtures to the specialist societies inviting them to become more actively involved. The BioMed Alliance that represents the European specialist societies now has a CME Experts Permanent Committee [16], which may be willing to engage in dialogue with the CME community. However, its credibility with the specialist societies may not improve until CME achieves comparable academic status to undergraduate medical education. Perhaps, only then will the societies let the CME community join their exclusive sailing club and berth in their well-appointed harbour.

REFERENCES

1. Sibley JC. A randomized trial of continuing medical education. *New England Journal of Medicine* 1982;306:511–515.
2. Berg AO. Does continuing medical education improve the quality of medical care? A look at the evidence. *The Journal of Family Practice* 1979;8(6):1171–1174.
3. Miller GE. Continuing education for what? *Journal of Medical Education* 1967;42(4):320–326. doi:10.1097/00001888-196704000-00003
4. Abrahamson S. Evaluation in continuing medical education. *JAMA* 1968;206(3):625–628. doi:10.1001/jama.1968.03150030081019
5. Bertram DA, Brooks-Bertram PA. The evaluation of continuing medical education: a literature review. *Health Education Monographs* 1977;5(4):330–362. doi:10.1177/109019817700500404
6. Fox RD. Discrepancy analysis in continuing medical education. *Mobius* 1983;3:37–44.
7. Knowles M. *The Adult Learner: A Neglected Species*. Gulf Publishing Company, Houston, Texas; 1973.
8. Festinger, L. *A Theory of Cognitive Dissonance*. Stanford University Press, California; 1957.
9. Hansen, E.J. Creating teachable moments... and making them last. *Innovative Higher Education* 1998;23:7–26. doi:10.1023/A:1022916412432
10. Haynes RB, Davis DA, McKibbon A, Tugwell P. A critical appraisal of the efficacy of continuing medical education. *JAMA* 1984;251:61–64.

11. Davis DA, Thomson MA, Oxman AD, Haynes RB. Evidence for the effectiveness of CME: A review of 50 randomized controlled trials. *JAMA* 1992;268(9):1111–1117. doi:10.1001/jama.1992.03490090053014

12. Davis D, O'Brien MAT, Freemantle N, Wolf FM, Mazmanian P, Taylor-Vaisey A. Impact of formal continuing medical education: Do conferences, workshops, rounds, and other traditional continuing education activities change physician behavior or health care outcomes? *JAMA* 1999;282(9):867–874. doi:10.1001/jama.282.9.867

13. Mansouri M, Lockyer J. A meta-analysis of continuing medical education effectiveness. *Journal of Continuing Education in the Health Professions* 2007;27(1):6–15. doi:10.1002/chp.88

14. Mazmanian PE, Davis DA, Galbraith R; American College of Chest Physicians Health and Science Policy Committee. Continuing medical education effect on clinical outcomes: effectiveness of continuing medical education: American College of Chest Physicians evidence-based educational guidelines. *Chest* 2009;135(3 Suppl):49S–55S. doi:10.1378/chest.08-2518.

15. Cervero RM, Gaines JK. The impact of CME on physician performance and patient health outcomes: An updated synthesis of systematic reviews. *Journal of Continuing Education in the Health Professions* 2015;35(2):131–138. doi:10.1002/chp.21290.

16. BioMed Alliance. https://www.biomedeurope.org/activities-medical-societies/cme-experts-permanent-committee.html

The Three Types of PPG

4

Medical practice is diverse and multi-faceted, and self-critical physicians will be aware of almost innumerable gaps in their daily practice. These would vary from diagnostic inadequacy to unpunctuality. In the context of CME, for practical purposes, it is reasonable to consider three types of PPG: deficiency, development and confidence [1].

DEFICIENCY GAP

This type of PPG occurs when there is a lack of physician knowledge, competence or performance. A knowledge gap affects individual physicians rather than large numbers, for example, when physicians are intending to prescribe a new drug for a patient, they may need to check whether the drug is likely to interact with any of the other drugs already prescribed. Similarly, physicians may become aware of a competence gap when they plan to perform a procedure such as a lumber puncture or chest intubation, which they do infrequently.

A performance gap is much more common and often occurs because of a barrier to the transfer of competence to performance. Such barriers are often cultural and liable to affect many physicians in whom particular cultural values are ingrained. Fifty years ago in the UK, tuberculosis clinics were being transformed into respiratory medicine clinics dealing with asthma, bronchitis and other chronic lung diseases. In many clinics, return patients had a routine chest X-ray at every visit, as had been the practice for TB patients. The physicians knew this was no longer necessary, but were reluctant to end a long-standing tradition. Newly appointed consultants in the 1980s had to indicate that this was a performance gap by showing the senior consultants that this practice was obsolete and was disappearing throughout the country. This is an example of a barrier between competence and performance. In this case, the barrier was the irrational and emotional attachment to a practice with which the seniors had grown up, but which had outlived its usefulness.

DOI: 10.1201/9781003270287-4

Much more recently, in an NHS Maternity Trust, high levels of stillbirths, neonatal and maternal deaths and birth injuries were reported [2]. The obstetricians and midwives had espoused a culture of "normal birth at almost any cost", which meant that the caesarean section rate was much lower than the national average and instrumental delivery was high. This is another example of poor performance related to outdated and old-fashioned cultural values.

Barriers to transfer of competence to performance may also happen because of system failure and may affect all the physicians and other healthcare professionals operating within the system. Between 2005 and 2009, the standard of care in an English general hospital was found to be appalling. The official report stated that "These failures were in part due to a focus on reaching targets, achieving financial balance and seeking foundation trust status at the cost of delivering acceptable standards of care". Staffing levels were too low, bullying and intimidation were common [3]. This was a system failure gap.

Misdiagnosis – The Clinical Acumen Gap

Not all performance gaps are due to barriers between competence and performance. Some do result from incompetence and of these, probably the most significant is misdiagnosis. Research into diagnostic failure is curiously sparse. In a Danish study, general practitioners (GPs) failed to make a specific diagnosis in 36% of patients with health problems [4]. In a large US outpatient study, the rate of diagnostic errors was in excess of 5% [5], although previous expert opinion estimates were 10%–15%. A survey of paediatricians found that more than half of them admitted to making diagnostic errors once or twice monthly [6]. An autopsy study of intensive treatment unit (ITU) patients found discordance between clinical and postmortem diagnoses of 19.8% [7]. On an anecdotal level, complaints about misdiagnosis by GPs and emergency medicine physicians are commonplace.

A Dutch study found that adverse events due to diagnostic failure were predominantly related to human error, either knowledge deficit or failure to apply knowledge correctly and contributed to patient death more frequently than other types of adverse events (29% vs. 7%) [8]. In a recent large US study, diagnostic error cases were found to comprise 28.7% of all US malpractice claims. Overall, 11,592 such cases were analysed and, of these, there were 7379 cases of high-severity harms, 53% of which led to death [9].

These data show the importance of misdiagnosis in contemporary healthcare. It may be the most important deficiency PPG, but this is not generally appreciated because CME aimed at deficiency PPGs is dominated by gaps in the treatment rather than the diagnosis of disease. This is a reflection of the disproportionate influence on CME content exerted by the drug industry, which tends to underestimate the importance of diagnosis in comparison with treatment. There is therefore a strong case for critically reviewing the provision of CME that concentrates on improving disease management with better drug treatment, while paying little attention to the problems in diagnosis of the disease. That said, we know that CME properly directed at the management and treatment of disease does work. Do we have any reason to believe that CME directed at better diagnosis would also work?

Diagnostic errors comprise three types: *no fault errors* where the presentation is atypical or inaccurately described, or when the disease is excessively rare or only recently discovered; *system errors* where working conditions are poor, physicians' workload is too high or communications are defective; and *cognitive errors* where data are wrongly interpreted, logic is faulty or biased reasoning is not recognised [10].

Of these, *no fault errors* may decrease as diseases become better understood. Previously, patients with Lyme disease were diagnosed as atypical rheumatoid arthritis. The easy availability of computed tomography (CT) and magnetic resonance imaging (MRI) scanners allows clinically occult pathologies to be detected, such as silent pancreatic or renal tumours. But rare diseases still occur and patients still misrepresent their symptoms and fail to keep appointments, so *no fault errors* will always be with us.

System errors once discovered should be amenable to repair. But all systems degrade over time and, like cars, need periodic servicing. When one faulty area in the system is corrected, the law of unintended consequences may allow another fault to develop. When scarce resources are used to fix one problem, others may persist unheeded for lack of funds. Nevertheless, many studies have examined how system improvements can help to reduce errors and delays in diagnosis. Most have been technology-driven based on algorithms for computerised trigger systems to alert physicians to laboratory or imaging results and to signal unwanted delays in the diagnostic process. An Australian systematic review of 26 studies of audit and communication strategies, which included nine randomised controlled trials (RCTs) found only limited evidence that the interventions improved diagnostic accuracy and reduced diagnostic delay [11].

To be considered to have *clinical acumen* is one of the most prized accolades physicians can receive from their peers. But it is seldom clear why some physicians have this elusive quality and others lack it. It does not correlate with intelligence or knowledge. Everyone knows the clever physician brimming over with facts, who is a useless doctor. The clue to solving this puzzle is to be found in the study of *cognitive errors*, which may occur because of stupidity, ignorance, failure to process and analyse data or bias.

Even if they have the necessary knowledge, stupid physicians will not be able to avoid cognitive errors. Lacking relevant knowledge, even clever physicians will not be able to consider possible diagnoses consistent with the facts of a case. Fortunately, most physicians are neither stupid nor ignorant.

Failure to process data may happen because physicians lack the drive or energy to marshall the facts of the case or having processed the data, they may not have the pattern recognition skills to suggest the diagnosis. As above, computerised trigger systems may help with data acquisition and processing. In radiology departments, educational team meetings and error documentation have been shown to reduce diagnostic error rates [11]. The proportion of cognitive errors attributable to these factors is not known, but when they have been excluded, those remaining will be due to bias. Experience suggests that physicians' decision-making is more susceptible to bias than that of airline pilots or civil engineers, but why should that be?

Bias is only important when the diagnosis is not obvious and so it matters little to an ophthalmologist dealing with a blind patient with advanced cataracts or to an orthopaedic surgeon with a patient who has fractured his femur. Perceptual specialties such as radiology and histopathology, which rely on visual interpretation, are said to have the lowest error rates [12]. However, in some specialties such as general practice and acute or emergency medicine, the diagnostic possibilities are huge, and patients are often seen with limited time to access and process information. In these circumstances of uncertainty and insufficient data, physicians resort to shortcuts known as heuristics to reach diagnoses. Heuristics are often oversimplified evaluations of situations based on experience or lessons learnt from others. Their use allows physicians to keep their heads above water by not having to reach every decision by laborious *a priori* reasoning. But the shortcut does not always work because, in some cases, the diagnosis is not as straightforward as it seems. The physician may not appreciate that because of one of the many biases that decision-makers are often unable to resist. The effect of the bias is to create a gap between analytical and heuristically determined behaviour resulting in a cognitive error and misdiagnosis [13,14].

There are now more than 30 documented biases. They include the following:

(i) *anchoring bias* when physicians may lock on to features in the initial presentation and be reluctant to adjust this impression in the light of later information.

(ii) *availability bias* makes physicians think of diagnoses that come readily to mind because of recent experience of similar cases.

(iii) *confirmation bias* encourages physicians uncritically to accept information that supports their first diagnosis rather than looking for evidence against it.

(iv) *omission bias* is the tendency towards inaction because physicians should *do no harm*.

(v) *overconfidence bias* induces physicians to act on inadequate data, intuition or hunches.

(vi) *premature closure bias* is the temptation to curtail the decision-making process before the diagnosis has been verified.

(vii) *search satisficing bias* is the universal tendency to call off a search once something has been found. Satisficing is a portmanteau word comprising satisfy and suffice [15].

(viii) *bias of sunk costs* makes physicians who have invested heavily in one diagnosis very reluctant to consider an alternative.

An increasing problem in modern medicine is *specialty bias* where specialists are blinkered towards any diagnoses not included within their specialty. For example, a cardiologist may see a patient with hysterical hyperventilation and will confidently exclude a cardiac cause but will have no interest in considering a non-cardiac cause for the disease. A young friend of the author was admitted to a surgical ward with left upper quadrant pain and fever. He had abdominal CT and ultrasound scans, and the surgeons were planning endoscopic procedures. When the author visited him, the pain was evidently pleuritic and the surgeons accepted the alternative diagnosis of viral pleurisy.

Much of the research has been directed at acute or emergency medicine where diagnosis is paramount. Physicians are encouraged to *think about their thinking*, a process called metacognition. This involves being able to stand apart from their thinking and analyse it, having previously learnt how the various biases can distort thinking [12,16,17]. Thoughtful physicians already do this instinctively when they discover that they have made a wrong diagnosis. Over time, iterative metacognitive analysis allows physicians to detect potential biases and resist them and at the same time develop pattern recognition associated with specific diagnoses. They also learn to look out for pitfalls in particular situations. For example, a physician was pleased to discover that an asthmatic patient's deterioration could be attributed to beta-blocker treatment for hypertension and further enquiry stopped because of the *satisficing bias*. If the physician had resisted the bias to stop, he would have discovered that the patient had also been prescribed beta-blocker eye drops for glaucoma. This bias is also the reason behind the trauma physician's aphorism, *the most commonly missed fracture is the second one* [18].

Some diagnoses need more than routine decision-making. Despite allowing for relevant biases, the diagnosis may remain obscure. When this happens, physicians' metacognition should extend beyond thinking about biases and turn to basic science. For example, respiratory physicians faced with a complex pulmonary pathological problem may draw on their pulmonary physiological knowledge to help them reach a diagnosis. Their understanding about gas exchange disturbance and resulting physiological responses may clear their minds. If this mental process is successful, they will be able to transfer it repeatedly to other clinical situations. But it is dependent on previously acquired knowledge, the *preparation for learning*, which should encourage them to brush up on their physiology and to persuade their colleagues to do likewise. This intellectual exercise allows the physicians to graduate from routine expertise to adaptive expertise, also known as Master Adaptive Learning [19,20].

The challenge for CME providers is whether they can help physicians to graduate from routine to adaptive expertise. The assumption is that this transition can be facilitated by physicians learning the precepts of metacognition. There is no evidence that this hypothesis has been rigorously tested, but it has been advocated [18,21], and it is suggested that CME should include the following:

(i) Physicians should make time for reflection when they stand back and consider whether their thinking about a case has been influenced by one of the biases. In an experimental setting, reflection has been found to be an effective debiasing agent [22]. Reflection should also encompass basic science.

(ii) Physicians should become familiar with the list of biases and practise debiasing strategies, such as always disciplining themselves to offer differential diagnoses.

(iii) Use of the *Five Whys* technique [23] where repeatedly asking *why* after sequential answers until no more answers are forth-coming can break through the biases and may reveal the cause of a difficult problem.

Many physicians will be sceptical about the value of reflective thinking in the process of diagnosis. *Which of you by taking thought can add one cubit unto his stature* [24]? Nevertheless, it may be a good discipline for physicians to question their first diagnosis in the knowledge of what can go wrong. At the very least these ideas could be tested by research studies.

This misdiagnosis gap is different from other deficiency gaps because CME does not ask physicians to change their therapeutic behaviour, but rather to change their diagnostic behaviour. To induce cognitive dissonance, physicians must be confronted by their diagnostic inadequacy, to admit to diagnostic failures which may have damaged their patients.

Many physicians would much rather forget about their missed or wrong diagnoses. Therefore, providers may find it difficult to create a teachable moment. To deal with physicians' sensitivity about their diagnostic prowess, or lack of it, might need an alternative approach. Perhaps, the problem should be viewed in the context of CPD rather than CME. This idea will be revisited in the chapter on CPD.

DEVELOPMENT GAP

This gap is common and happens when physicians fail to keep up to date. Almost 40 years ago, respiratory physicians in a large teaching hospital became aware of a high readmission rate of patients with uncontrolled asthma. They conducted a prospective audit and found that patients discharged from wards with no respiratory physicians were more likely to be readmitted to the hospital than patients discharged from wards with respiratory input. They found that the readmitted patients had not had their inhaled steroid therapy optimised and explained to them before their recent discharge. This was a development PPG because the physicians in the non-respiratory wards were not aware that inhaled steroids were revolutionising asthma treatment when used correctly. On the other hand, the respiratory physicians, aware of this important development, had suspected the presence of the gap in the general wards [25].

When a drug company has a new drug that it wants to promote, it may approach a commercial CME provider in order to support a CME intervention designed to fill a development PPG. In 2019, a US commercial provider won the Innovative Format Award from the *Alliance for Continuing Education in the Health Professions* for a gamification programme on the treatment of rheumatoid arthritis with a kinase inhibitor. This drug was produced by Pfizer, which had supported the study [26]. Physicians do well to be wary of CME for development PPGs, which may be tackled better by discussion among colleagues and reference to specialist society guidelines.

The manner of learning about a new drug or technique depends on the type of learner. If the learners are trainees, the education will just be added to their curriculum. Trainees are programmed to learn what is offered to them. The history of CME shows that this is not true for established physicians who must be predisposed to learn in a teachable moment. The relevance of the development gap to their practice must be made evident to them. Therefore, the education committees of specialist societies should be prepared to deliver education on the same subject in two different ways.

CONFIDENCE GAP

This gap happens when physicians have become unsure that "what they are doing" is still "what they should be doing" and has not become out of date because of new developments. Such gaps do not make physicians as uncomfortable as deficiency gaps, but may be the reason that physicians attend lectures where confidence in their current practice is reinforced. This may be a justification for state-of-the-art lectures at the annual congresses of specialist societies on the grounds that they are filling confidence gaps. This is much less trouble than discovering and analysing a deficiency PPG and customising CME to repair it.

In general, in this port-of-call, physicians are reminded that understanding practice gaps is the essential tool they need to maintain and develop their continuing education.

REFERENCES

1. Adapted from Moore DE. *Personal Communication.* 2020
2. Dyer C. Maternity care: services across England require "immediate and essential actions". *BMJ* 2020;371:m4797.
3. Francis R. Mid Staffordshire NHS Foundation Trust Public Inquiry 2013 https://webarchive.nationalarchives.gov.uk/ukgwa/20150407084231/http:/www.midstaffspublicinquiry.com/report
4. Rosendal M, Carlsen AH, Rask MT, Moth G. Symptoms as the main problem in primary care: A cross-sectional study of frequency and characteristics. *Scandinavian Journal of Primary Health Care* 2015 Jun;33(2):91–99. doi:10.31 09/02813432.2015.1030166.
5. Singh H, Meyer AND, Thomas EJ The frequency of diagnostic errors in outpatient care: Estimations from three large observational studies involving US adult populations *BMJ Quality & Safety* 2014;23:727–731.
6. Singh H, Thomas EJ, Wilson L, Kelly PA, Pietz K, Elkeeb D, Singhal G. Errors of diagnosis in pediatric practice: a multisite survey. *Pediatrics* 2010;126(1):70–79. doi: 10.1542/peds.2009-3218.
7. Tai DY, El-Bilbeisi H, Tewari S, Mascha EJ, Wiedemann HP, Arroliga AC. A study of consecutive autopsies in a medical ICU: a comparison of clinical cause of death and autopsy diagnosis. *Chest* 2001;119(2):530–536. doi: 10.1378/chest.119.2.530.

8. Zwaan L, de Bruijne M, Wagner C, et al. Patient record review of the incidence, consequences, and causes of diagnostic adverse events. *Archives of Internal Medicine* 2010;170(12):1015–1021. doi:10.1001/archinternmed.2010.146

9. Newman-Toker DE, Schaffer AC, Yu-Moe CW, Nassery N, Saber Tehrani AS, Clemens GD, Wang Z, Zhu Y, Fanai M, Siegal D. Serious misdiagnosis-related harms in malpractice claims: The "Big Three" – vascular events, infections, and cancers. *Diagnosis (Berl).* 2019;6(3):227–240. doi: 10.1515/dx-2019-0019.

10. Graber M, Gordon R, Franklin N. Reducing diagnostic errors in medicine: What's the goal? *Academic Medicine* 2002;77(10):981–992. doi: 10.1097/00001888-200210000-00009.

11. Abimanyi-Ochom J, Bohingamu Mudiyanselage S. Catchpool M. Firipis M, Wanni Arachchige Dona S, Watts J. Strategies to reduce diagnostic errors: A systematic review. *BMC Medical Informatics and Decision Making* 2019;19:174. doi:10.1186/s12911-019-0901-1

12. Berner ES, Graber ML. Overconfidence as a cause of diagnostic error in medicine. *American Journal of Medicine* 2008;121(5A):S2–S23.

13. Croskerry P. The importance of cognitive errors in diagnosis and strategies to minimize them. *Academic Medicine* 2003;78(8):775–780. doi: 10.1097/00001888-200308000-00003.

14. O'Sullivan ED, Schofield SJ. Cognitive bias in clinical medicine. *Journal of the Royal College of Physicians of Edinburgh* 2018;48:225–232. doi:10.4997/JRCPE.2018.306

15. https://en.wikipedia.org/wiki/Satisficing

16. Hamm RM. Figure and ground in physician misdiagnosis: Metacognition and diagnostic norms. *Diagnosis (Berl)* 2014;1(1):29–33. doi:10.1515/dx-2013-0019

17. Scott IA, Crock C. Diagnostic error: Incidence, impacts, causes and preventive strategies. *Medical Journal of Australia* 2020;213:302–305. doi:10.5694/mja2.50771

18. Croskerry P. Adaptive expertise in medical decision making. *Medical Teacher* 2018;40(8):803–808. doi:10.1080/0142159X.2018.1484898

19. Cutrer WB, Miller B, Pusic MV, Mejicano G, Mangrulkar RS, Gruppen LD, Hawkins RE, Skochelak SE, Moore DE Jr. Fostering the development of master adaptive learners: A conceptual model to guide skill acquisition in medical education. *Academic Medicine* 2017;92(1):70–75. doi:10.1097/ACM.0000000000001323

20. Mylopoulos M, Brydges R, Woods NN, Manzone J, Schwartz DL. Preparation for future learning: A missing competency in health professions education? *Medical Education* 2016 Jan;50(1):115–123. doi:10.1111/medu.12893

21. Colbert CY, Graham L, West C, White BA, Arroliga AC, Myers JD, Ogden PE, Archer J, Mohammad ZT, Clark J. Teaching metacognitive skills: Helping your physician trainees in the quest to 'know what they don't know'. *American Journal of Medicine* 2015;128(3):318–324. doi:10.1016/j.amjmed.2014.11.001

22. Mamede S, van Gog T, van den Berge K, et al. Effect of availability bias and reflective reasoning on diagnostic accuracy among internal medicine residents. *JAMA* 2010;304(11):1198–1203. doi:10.1001/jama.2010.1276

23. Serrat O. *The Five Whys Technique.* Asian Development Bank, Washington, DC; 2010. https://www.researchgate.net/publication/318013490_The_Five_Whys_Technique
24. Matthew cha. 6, v. 27. *King James Bible* London, 1611.
25. Bucknall CE, Robertson C, Moran F, Stevenson RD. Differences in hospital asthma management. *Lancet* 1988;i:748–750.
26. Do You Know JAK? Effectively Using Gamification for CME/CPD. 2019. http://almanac.acehp.org/p/bl/et/blogid=2&blogaid=411

Gap Discovery and Analysis

5

Gap discovery is complex and multi-layered. Individual countries should consider a hierarchical structure by which gaps are discovered, extending from the lowest level of a single physician to the highest level of their national medical authorities. Once discovered, a PPG must be analysed to find out its cause. It is helpful to relate the cause to the relevant level on Moore's Pyramid of Outcomes (Figure 5.1), because this helps the CME planner to design the most appropriate type of reparative CME. This approach is now almost universally accepted as a result of Don Moore's seminal paper published in 2009 [1].

PHYSICIAN LEVEL

Every time a physician faces a clinical situation where he does not know what to do, he exposes a PPG between what he knows and what he should know. Analysis shows that these PPGs are usually level 3, learning or knowledge gaps, or level 4, competence gaps. A physician often reacts to these gaps by using informal CME when he takes advice from a colleague (corridor consult) or repairs his knowledge gap by accessing UpToDate® or a specialist society website on his mobile phone. This is the most common and simplest type of gap discovery and happens so naturally that physicians are not aware that they are engaging in CME because the transaction is so informal.

The fly in the ointment is that physicians cannot be trusted to recognise their own PPGs and this is particularly true for physicians who perform less well than their peers [2]. This is one of the many reasons why no physician should be an island and that performance should be externally assessed. This can be done by a process of annual appraisal including multi-source feedback, which is now established in the UK and contributes to physician revalidation every 5 years.

DOI: 10.1201/9781003270287-5

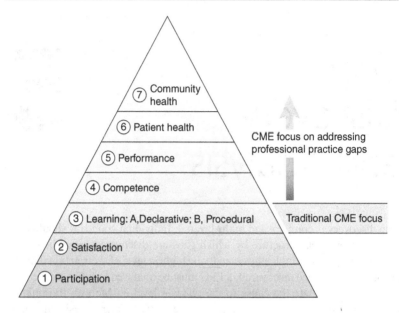

FIGURE 5.1   Moore's CME Outcomes Pyramid.

HOSPITAL LEVEL

Most North American hospitals have dedicated education departments, which include responsibility for CME and CPD, although they have been decreasing in number because of paperwork and cost. In Europe, these are the exception rather than the rule. Such departments organise courses, webinars, meetings with experts and skills workshops. In addition, they often have responsibility for undergraduate and graduate education, in which case andragogy must hold its own against pedagogy.

Ideally, the CME Department would be sensible of its responsibility actively to search for PPGs. This should feed off the Quality Improvement (QI) activities that hospitals are required to set up and which should be aware of those aspects of hospital life where quality has been found wanting [3]. For example the microbiology department will know whether the hospital's level of hospital-acquired infections is above or below the national average. Cooperation between the CME and QI departments should allow PPGs to be identified and analysed. In most cases, the PPG will relate to a hospital unit or team, but on occasions, it will relate to an individual physician whose performance has been questioned. These PPGs will usually be level 4, competence, or level 5, performance, and their repair will require some kind of formal CME intervention.

SPECIALIST LEVEL

All medical specialties have national and international societies, which have many functions, not least of which is the provision of CME to their members. The non-medical staff of the societies are often aware of the developments in modern CME, but the same is not true for the medical staff who are usually elected to serve on the education committee for a limited time, having had no previous experience of CME. To people such as these, the idea that CME is quite different from undergraduate or graduate education often comes as a surprise.

Like hospital CME departments, the society CME committees should look for PPGs in their specialty practice. Usually, this has meant carrying out an audit of the management of specific diseases. In 2013, the European Respiratory Society (ERS) reported on the design of an audit into the management and outcome of exacerbations of chronic obstructive pulmonary disease. They conducted a prospective non-interventional cohort trial in two phases in 13 countries involving 422 hospitals [4]. PPGs were discovered, for example, almost 20% of patients did not have blood gas analysis on admission [5], and this allowed the ERS to design CME aimed at improving the management of such patients. This undertaking depleted ERS financial resources and needed considerable time and effort to produce information on PPGs that turned out to be predictable and unexciting. The ERS is unlikely to embark on a similar audit project without greater expectation of a more significant outcome.

Fortunately, digitisation of clinical information is becoming established in many countries. NHS Digital [6], UK Biobank [7], Statewide Health Information Network for New York [8] and the developing European Electronic Health Records Network [9,10] will make it possible for researchers to interrogate *big data*, and there may be no need to carry out cumbersome, large-scale audits in the future. Such interrogation is easier said than done and is best achieved by the new specialty of Healthcare Data Scientists who are trained in mathematics, statistics, epidemiology and informatics[11,12]. The gap component described as "what is" is derived from analysis of *big data*. The full definition of a gap also needs the other component known as "what should be". This is available from standards of care published by specialist societies or from journals such as *BMJ Best Practice*.

Most gap discovery and analysis (needs assessment) have concentrated on disease management, but the recent interest in decision theory and misdiagnosis discussed in the last chapter should prompt societies to investigate PPGs in the diagnostic competence of their members. Diagnostic accuracy may not be specifically documented in health records, but the time between the presenting symptoms and reaching the definitive diagnosis is a surrogate for diagnostic competence. For example, when several months elapse between presentation with iron-deficiency anaemia and the discovery of colon cancer, investigation into diagnostic competence would be justified.

Some gaps or discrepancies make their discovery easy when they are taken up by the press and social media. For example, many physicians feel that the behaviour of those involved in the management of gender dysphoria is far removed from an acceptable standard and therefore represents a practice gap [13]. It is not clear whether this is a purely medical problem or whether cultural or societal influences may also be relevant. In this case, discovery of the PPG is easy, but analysis to find its cause would be fraught with difficulty.

At a practical level, a specialist society or a drug firm may define a PPG and subsequently engage the services of a professional provider to plan and design the CME. For the CME to be acceptable for accreditation, the supporting organisation must not influence the work of the provider. CME provided in this way should be of good quality, because independent providers are professional educators whose business is to deliver CME according to the rules. That said, many of the larger drug firms have CME departments that organise their Requests For Proposals (RFPs) directed at professional providers. There is often tension between the two when the drug firm CME experts are critical of the expertise of the provider.

In many chronic diseases, there are now patient organisations for support, advocacy and promotion of research. These should cooperate with the society CME committees in PPG discovery and analysis. Too often, societies engage with patient groups in a spirit of tokenism which is ill-advised because they often have first-hand experience of gaps from the other side of the fence.

NATIONAL NON-SPECIALIST LEVEL

There are gaps that transcend specialist practice and affect healthcare across the length and breadth of a country. Analysis of these PPGs should be the business of national medical associations, such as the Royal Colleges in the UK and Canada, independent charitable organisations such as the King's Fund in the UK [14], Centers for Medicare and Medicaid Services in the US and the German Medical Association (Bundesärztekammer), and these PPGs will usually relate to levels 6 and 7. Like specialist societies, these organisations should know how to interrogate *big data*.

Two examples include opioid abuse where unscrupulous drug firms broadcast false assurances about the use of their analgesics and CME to address this problem has been necessary, and secondly antibiotic resistance, where ongoing CME intervention is needed to remind physicians to prescribe antibiotics prudently. Delay in radiological investigation because of too few CT or MRI scanners is a system failure attributable to management decisions rather than poor physician performance and so falls out with the scope of CME. Nevertheless, the organisation that discovered the gap has a responsibility to apprise management of it.

An important PPG in this category relates to the damage to quality of life because of too active care of patients at the end-of-life or suffering from dementia. Similar questions are asked about active treatment for babies with gross birth defects. In these cases, the cause of the gap is cultural rather than educational deficit. In a previous, less secular age, active treatment in such patients was discouraged and doctors believed that "pneumonia was the old man's friend". Now demented patients with pneumonia are admitted to hospitals from care homes and treated with intravenous antibiotics.

The idea that death might be welcomed in such circumstances is no longer mentioned in polite society. In an animal species with no natural predator, this change in our attitude to death makes little sense, but is nevertheless increasingly prevalent and is accepted by many, especially younger physicians. For the moment, the medical establishment still quietly favours the old philosophy and must decide whether to defend it or to follow the modern trend. If it opts to resist, it should design CME for its own younger members to persuade them that prolongation of life at almost any cost is foolish, cruel and against society's long-term interests.

A new PPG has become evident during the COVID pandemic. Previously, physicians managed obese patients by forcefully explaining the hazards of obesity and advocating dietary and exercise advice. This approach was criticised as being *fat shaming* by a generation programmed to being easily offended and physicians largely stopped upbraiding patients for their obesity.

Recent evidence from the World Obesity Federation shows that of the 2.5 million COVID deaths reported by the end of February 2021, 2.2 million were in countries where over half the population is classified as overweight [15]. This knowledge challenges current acceptance by physicians of the right to be obese. Failure to resist and criticise the epidemic of obesity can be regarded as a PPG because the susceptibility of obese people to coronavirus contributes to its spreading in the population. This is another example of a cultural factor causing a PPG.

National healthcare organisations have a responsibility to arrange CME to counter PPGs, which are related to cultural influences. Ideally, the CME should be interprofessional so that the treatment advice can be delivered on a broad front. Unfortunately, in the case of obesity, many of the healthcare professionals are themselves afflicted by the problem.

As our voyage leaves this harbour, the take-home message is that the primary responsibility for finding and investigating PPGs rests with the healthcare professionals themselves and their professional bodies and not with managers, bureaucrats, drug firms and politicians.

REFERENCES

1. Moore DE, Green JS, Gallis HA. Achieving the desired results and improved outcomes: Integrating planning and assessment throughout learning activities. *Journal of Continuing Education in the Health Professions* 2009;29(1):1–15.
2. Davis DA, Mazmanian PE, Fordis M, Van Harrison R, Thorpe KE, Perrier L. Accuracy of physician self-assessment compared with observed measures of competence: a systematic review. *JAMA* 2006;296(9):1094–1102. doi:10.1001/jama.296.9.1094
3. Archibald D, Burns JK, Fitzgerald, M, Merkley VF. Aligning practice data and institution-specific CPD: Medical quality management as the driver for an eLearning development process. *Journal of European CME* 2020;9:1. doi:10.1 080/21614083.2020.1754120
4. López-Campos JL, Hartl S, Pozo-Rodriguez FC, Roberts M. (on behalf of the European COPD Audit team). European COPD audit: Design, organisation of work and methodology. *European Respiratory Journal* 2013;41:270–276. doi:10.1183/09031936.00021812
5. Hartl S, Lopez-Campos JL, Pozo-Rodriguez F, Castro-Acosta A, Studnicka M, Kaiser B, Roberts CM. Risk of death and readmission of hospital-admitted COPD exacerbations: European COPD audit. *European Respiratory Journal* 2016;47(1):113–121. doi:10.1183/13993003.01391–2014
6. NHS digital. https://digital.nhs.uk/
7. UK Biobank. http://www.ukbiobank.ac.uk/
8. Statewide Health Information Network for New York. 2006. https://www.nyehealth.org/shin-ny/what-is-the-shin-ny/
9. European electronic health records network. https://ec.europa.eu/health/sites/health/files/ehealth/docs/laws_report_recommendations_en.pdf
10. Exchange of electronic health records across the EU. https://digital-strategy.ec.europa.eu/en/policies/electronic-health-records
11. Meyer MA. Healthcare data scientist qualifications, skills, and job focus: a content analysis of job postings. *Journal of the American Medical Informatics Association* 2019;26(5):383–391. doi: 10.1093/jamia/ocy181
12. MSc Health Data Science. https://www.lshtm.ac.uk/study/courses/masters-degrees/health-data-science
13. Bell-v-Tavistock-Judgment. 2020. https://www.judiciary.uk/wp-content/uploads/2020/12/Bell-v-Tavistock-Judgment.pdf
14. King's Fund. https://www.kingsfund.org.uk/about-us
15. World Obesity Federation. https://www.worldobesity.org

CME Provision

6

CME providers comprise national and international specialist societies, medical associations, medical schools, hospitals and commercial organisations. Pharmaceutical companies may facilitate CME but not provide it, although in some countries in Latin America, industry-funded CME is accredited. There are three main types of CME provision – workplace informal, external formal and external informal.

WORKPLACE INFORMAL CME

mHealth – Self-Directed Point-of-Care CME

eHealth encompasses all electronic technologies in healthcare. Those directed towards education are described as eLearning, which includes live interactive media such as webinars and enduring materials accessible anywhere and at any time. Live internet activities and enduring materials accessed by mobile devices fall into the category of mobile health or mHealth, defined by the World Health Organisation as "medical and public health practice supported by mobile devices, such as mobile phones, patient monitoring devices, personal digital assistants (PDAs), and other wireless devices".

mHealth is a rapidly growing industry increasingly used by patients to help manage their diseases. In 2012, there were approximately 40,000 mobile device applications (apps) related to health [1]. mHealth includes telemedicine, electronic health records, disease monitoring, patient appointments and reminders. mHealth enduring materials are the basis for self-directed point-of-care CME when physicians use their mobile phones or smart watches to access medical databases at the bedside or in the clinic. Examples of these resources include UpToDate [2], a comprehensive clinical decision support resource; Edocate [3], a virtual patient simulation platform; ONCOassist [4], a decision support app in oncology; and YouTube videos or other software platforms created by specialist societies or commercial providers. When physicians use mHealth for point-of-care CME, they are of course repairing PPGs that they have discovered themselves.

It is difficult to appreciate the enormity of this workplace CME revolution that has been fuelled by the happy coincidence of universal mobile phone dependency and the availability of the above electronic databases. The COVID pandemic has brought this to light. Between January and August 2020, there were over 7.5 million COVID point-of-care CME searches registered by UpToDate. This kind of CME is a form of micro-learning which has been used in industry for decades [5–7].

CME is more effective when it includes repetition and reinforcement [8]. Therefore, point-of-care CME episodes should be recorded by the learner with notes on resulting practice change and proposed review after a time interval. Learners claim credits in some countries for engaging in point-of-care CME. UpToDate awards US credits for each completed learning cycle, which comprises documenting the clinical question, identifying the topics and reflecting on the application of findings to practice.

Multi-Disciplinary Team Meetings (MDTMs)

Over the past 50 years, the organisation of healthcare has changed radically. Previously, each of the professions, medicine, nursing, pharmacy and physiotherapy, had clearly defined hierarchical structures both of themselves and in relation to others. In medicine, the various disciplines interacted with one another on personal levels, but remained professionally distinct and separate.

There was general formality of address and first names were used sparingly. The weaknesses of this system gradually became evident, as medicine became more complex and the demands on it increased. Team working was seen to be effective and became socially and professionally acceptable, although old habits die hard. A nurse who worked with the author was heard to say "Hell will freeze over before I call him Robin".

These changes in professional attitudes are reflected in the development of the Multi-Disciplinary Team Meeting (MDTM) but also in the Patient Care Conference and Patient Case Discussion, all of which have become increasingly important features of hospital life. Although MDTMs were created primarily to improve patient management, it was gradually appreciated that they were providing surprisingly effective, informal CME. This discovery is supported by recent academic interest in the importance of dialogue in bridging sub-cultures in organisational learning [8]. As medicine has become increasingly complex, people from different, but inter-dependent disciplines have created communities of practice, one of which has been described as the knowledge-building community that is particularly aimed at the learning of knowledge [9].

In a study on information sharing in MDTMs, the *community of interaction* that was demonstrated in meetings contributes to the amplification and development of new knowledge and can be regarded as an important mechanism for organisational learning [10]. Participants were found to learn not only from others but also from their own contributions when the need to articulate information develops their own understanding. Educational gain from MDTMs was proportional to the level of contribution by the participants.

The interactivity of MDTMs furnishes participants with feedback, an essential component of learning. Within the confines of their own disciplines, clinicians are often protected from criticism often because juniors are unwilling to embarrass their elders. In MDTMs, clinical decisions and actions are exposed to peer review, which may be more objective and less charitable. Did the physician order the right investigations? Was the biopsy material adequate? Did the radiologist define the extent and operability of the lesion? Were the margins of the excised tissue free of tumour? Was the delay in diagnosis acceptable?

Most MDTMs will have several associated specialist societies. For example, a lung cancer MDTM will relate to societies for thoracic surgery, respiratory medicine, oncology, radiology and pathology. It is disappointing that such societies at present take little interest in the education of their members while attending MDTMs. There is no published research on the CME potential of MDTMs. Ideally, societies should both encourage such research and help their members to conduct the MDTMs in such a way as to optimise their educational value.

A senior physician, or a health professional with an interest in CME, should be nominated as the educational supervisor, and should keep an attendance record, compile a list of the clinical problems discussed and indicate when the outcomes might lead to practice change. The supervisor should ensure that proceedings are not dominated by any one physician, limit the number of cases discussed and encourage Q&A. Discussion need not involve all patients seen in the previous week, but should focus on those who are problematic. In some cases, it may be possible for problems requiring decisions to be circulated to the participants before the meeting. The supervisor should submit regular reports to the CME committees of the specialist societies.

In the future, MDTMs may be complemented by interprofessional team meetings that allow opportunities for informal interprofessional learning (IPL) in contrast to the more formal structured interprofessional education (IPE). A recent Australian study showed that interprofessional team meetings provided a practical, time-efficient and relevant means for IPL [11]. Teams were recruited comprising physicians, nurses and at least one other profession for both in- and out-patient team meetings. It was evident that informal learning was generally unexpected in the workplace and it was suggested that the learning opportunities should be emphasised. Underlying tensions between the physicians and other health professionals and an *us and them* attitude were observed, although this was less evident in younger team members. Considering the precedent of the success of MDTMs, it is likely that IPL meetings will also become established features of modern healthcare, but they may need encouragement from hospital CME or QI departments.

The defining feature of informal CME is that it is a response to the immediate and obvious need of physicians to find a solution to a clinical problem. In other words, the physicians are aware of the PPG which renders them cognitively dissonant, thereby creating a teachable moment for accessible workplace CME. Workplace CME by its nature involves limited numbers of physicians for individual educational interventions.

For years, the CME community was riven by doubts that formal CME may not affect physicians' performance and patient health. To everyone's relief, their doubts were resolved by the paper from Cervero and Gaines [12]. So great was the preoccupation with this issue that the mushroom growth of point-of-care CME and MDTMs went almost unnoticed. Informal CME had stolen a march on its formal partner and has added a new and exciting dimension to the CME world. Looking up a text-book in the coffee room after the ward round is a thing of the past.

EXTERNAL FORMAL CME

Live Event

This was the main type of CME until the explosion of informal, workplace CME along with external use of enduring materials. It comprises courses, annual congresses and regularly scheduled series. Previously, most discrepancies or PPGs were addressed by some form of live event, whereas now, many PPGs in levels 3 and 4 are being repaired by informal CME. As noted previously, many gaps, particularly in the higher levels, may not be immediately evident to physicians and therefore not amenable to informal, workplace CME. Such gaps usually need one of the types of formal CME, among which the live event is still popular because it lends itself to interactivity with face-to-face learner involvement. When CME planners are dealing with higher-level PPGs, they may be said to be engaged in the *ascent to the summit of the*

CME pyramid [13]. After the pyramid level is confirmed, usually 5, 6 or 7, the planner must then determine whether lack of knowledge, competence or performance is the cause of the gap. Armed with this information, the planner should attempt backwards planning, as described by Moore and colleagues, to allow the provider to customise the CME so that it is appropriate for the desired outcome level [14].

Backwards Planning

After discovery and analysis of a patient health PPG (level 6), the CME planner must descend Moore's pyramid step-wise starting from performance level 5 to find out if the patient health deficit was due to inadequate clinical performance (Figure 6.1). If performance appears to have been satisfactory, sociological, cultural or environmental influences on patient behaviour are likely. If performance is sub-optimal, the planner must descend the pyramid to competence level 4 to assess whether it is adequate. If clinical competence

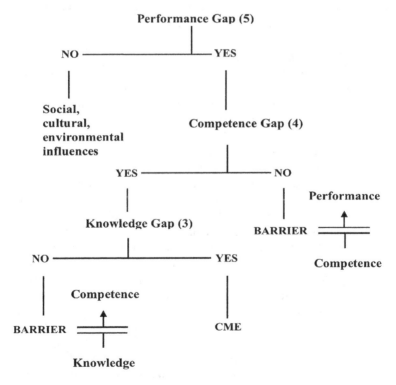

FIGURE 6.1 Backwards planning.

appears to have been satisfactory, a barrier blocking transfer of competence to performance should be suspected and sought. If competence is found not to have been satisfactory, the planner must descend again to learning or knowledge level 3. If knowledge appears to have been adequate, the planner must look for deficiency in the training of practical skills and offer suitable remedial education. If knowledge is found to have been inadequate, the planner should design appropriate didactic education, although in modern medical practice, this is becoming less common, partly because of the success of informal workplace CME.

Implementation

Having defined and analysed the PPG and applied this knowledge to enable backwards planning, the planner must then implement the educational objectives. In the pre-COVID era, for live events, Moore has recommended using a framework comprising three components, predisposing – enabling – reinforcing, reviewed recently by Porter [15]. During the COVID era, live events were replaced by virtual events, but since we can hope for the return of live events, it is reasonable to consider Moore's recommendations in some detail.

a. Predisposing
   The provider exploits physicians' discomfort when they learn of the PPG to create a teachable moment which renders them receptive to the CME intervention. This is done by email messages, hospital intranet or participation in a scenario.

b. Enabling
   Physicians should be enabled to implement what they have learnt guided by Merrill's principles of instruction [16]. The provider should try to make the educational material as authentic and realistic as possible. The learners' existing knowledge should be brought to the surface and activated as a foundation for the addition of new knowledge. To do this, learners should be encouraged to recall previous experiences that yielded knowledge of the same kind as the new knowledge. They must not just be told the new knowledge; it must be demonstrated to them possibly in a multimedia presentation. Having been exposed to it, the learners should apply the new knowledge themselves in an attempt to solve a real-life problem perhaps by taking part in a scenario, followed by feedback dialogue from experts. This last is also known as *formative assessment* or *assessment for learning* [17] and describes the interaction between learner and teacher which augments the quality of the education.

c. Reinforcing

Providers seek to remind learners of what they have learnt by means of repeated messages on mobile devices and inquiries into the degree of behaviour change and its duration. Reinforcement of knowledge and competence strengthens the confidence of learners in what they have learnt, thereby making behaviour change more likely [18].

This approach may seem excessively academic and theoretical, but high-level CME involves sociological and philosophical concepts such as the cost of saving lives, the comparative value of different lives, the acceptance of death and cultural factors inimical to health. Learners do not find this easy and providers must be sensible of ingrained and deeply rooted prejudices.

Performance Improvement CME (PI CME)

This is a special category of CME set up to direct CME towards outcomes and it consists of three stages:

a. assessment of clinical practice using identified evidence-based performance measures and identification of PPGs;
b. design and implementation of a suitable educational intervention;
c. re-evaluation of those performance measures to gauge improvement.

The American Medical Association and the American Academy of Family Physicians approved the standards for PI CME in 2004. It seemed like a good idea at the time, but has not taken off. In 2013, it comprised 0.4% of total ACCME activities of 138,196, and in 2019, it had fallen to 0.3% of 188,992 total activities [19,20]. It may yet become more popular, but it is perhaps seen as overly contrived.

eLearning

a. Enduring materials

Formal eLearning comes in many guises. It began as digital education limited to single computers loaded with a CD-ROM. Now it is based on the internet and includes enduring material comprising interactive case-based and text-based activities, YouTube videos, multi-media activities, gamification [21], virtual patient simulations [22], branching scenarios and archived webcasts.

The increase in usage of internet enduring materials in the US has been staggering. Between 2013 and 2019, annual enduring material activities rose from 19,068 to 49,431, physician interactions from 3,378,806 to 5,647,199 and non-physician interactions from 5,130,125 to 13,579,407. In 2019, there were more physician and other learner interactions in internet enduring materials than for any other educational modality [19,20].

Learners can access internet enduring materials at any time and at any place. First they become aware of a PPG. Then they search the internet to find relevant CME. To be suitable, the CME should be interactive with the computer replacing the human teacher in various settings, for example, in real-time chat, or two way audio/text/video-conferencing. Synchronous is preferable to asynchronous interaction although more difficult to implement, and repetition should always be possible by accessing the CME website later. Providers may offer a pre-test to learners with a post-test after the CME and award of credits is dependent on an acceptable post-test result.

When criteria such as these are met, internet-based learning results in strongly positive effects in knowledge, skills and practice behaviours compared to non-intervention. These effects are of course much less marked when compared with traditional CME methods [23,24]. Technology-enhanced simulation training has been shown to result in marked effects on knowledge, skills and behaviours with lesser effects on patient health [25]. Mastery learning can be applied to simulation-based medical education (SBME) in which learners may not proceed to the next stage until they have mastered the preceding one. When compared with non-mastery SBME, this added sophistication was associated with large benefit in skills, but took more time [26].

In an important comparative study of 114 internet CME activities, delivered to a large group of practising physicians, clinical case vignettes were presented after the CME to the participants and to a control group of non-participants, and then evidence-based clinical decisions were compared between the two groups. The participants in the CME were found to have an almost 50% greater likelihood of making clinical choices based on evidence [27].

b. Virtual live events

In the COVID era, specialist societies have replaced their annual congresses and other events with live webcasts of virtual meetings and conferences often using the Zoom platform. Initially, there were hour-long sessions with the faculty or main speaker holding the floor for 30 or 45 minutes followed by Q&A. Gradually, upon the instigation of the participants, the initial presentation has been progressively shortened and in some cases completely replaced by Q&A. Participants may be informed of any necessary reading beforehand and supplied with appropriate links. As the technology has become more sophisticated, parallel break-out sessions have followed plenary sessions, with each electing a rapporteur who will discuss the views of the break-out sessions at a subsequent review plenary. The sessions may be recorded and accessed from the society website as archived webcasts of enduring material.

In other words, the formal CME of the conference, often with limited learner involvement, has been transformed into a more interactive, probably more effective and certainly much cheaper form of CME. Lastly, for outcome assessment, reflections of participants can easily be recorded, thereby facilitating the award of credits by the provider.

Hybrid Events

The success of virtual live events during COVID makes it unlikely that post-COVID, live events will just pick up where they left off. Many organisations will be unwilling to pay for their members to attend expensive live events when virtual events have been so popular and so heavily subscribed. Nevertheless, the organisers of an event do want to meet one another in the flesh, partly for social reasons but also to participate in live panel discussions. Therefore, hybrid events will be arranged where key personnel will gather together in a place with unlimited internet access which will function as the operational hub of the event.

Interprofessional Continuing Education

In recent years, the CME community has sought to establish Interprofessional Continuing Education (IPCE) in the healthcare professions. In the US, the Institute of Medicine identified the importance of working in interprofessional teams and called on accreditors, licensing and certifying bodies to use their authority to leverage necessary organisational changes [28]. Towards that end, three of the national accreditors in medicine, nursing and pharmacy have collaborated to create a unified accreditation system to incentivise the development of IPCE [29].

We can consider IPE to have been the progenitor of IPCE and both to represent formal structured education in contrast to the more informal IPL.

There have now been many reports of IPE, recently analysed by Reeves and colleagues [30] who carried out a systematic review of 46 studies. They were descriptive rather than RCTs and outcomes were largely based on self-reporting. The studies were heterogeneous with many involving undergraduates, graduates and primary care physicians. A minority dealt with in-service CME. As noted above with IPL, there were problems with negative professional stereotyping, but overall the outcomes were considered positive.

Not all PPGs are suitable for repair by IPCE. Some relate solely to physicians' practice and probably some are confined to nursing or pharmaceutical behaviours. CME planners should design CME for the appropriate audience, be it mono-, bi- or multi-professional. The gaps where all the health professions are involved are those where cultural factors are important. These include end-of-life care, approach to dementia, indications for resuscitation, smoking, alcoholism, drug addiction, obesity, epidemics, pandemics and vaccination. All of these pose difficult questions for us to answer. How do we reconcile human rights with dangers to public health? To what extent should family members influence treatment of our patients? How do we prioritise care of COVID patients in relation to cancer patients? What do we say to anti-vaxxers?

It must be right for healthcare professions to tackle these issues together. It is likely that different opinions will be held by the different professions, but society will be best served if the disparate views can be harmonised into a consensus. This is a major challenge to the CME planners of the individual professions.

EXTERNAL INFORMAL CME

In the pre-COVID era, physicians from different hospitals in the area would meet together perhaps monthly, for case presentations and research reports, often in late afternoon and followed by eating and drinking in the evening. In recent years, attendance at such meetings has been declining perhaps because of increased pressure of work and more demanding family obligations. They stopped completely during COVID. However, there are now anecdotal reports that the webinar concept underpinning live formal CME is increasingly being used to breathe life back into external informal CME meetings. These are now happening in the shape of small group virtual meetings, but sadly without the face-to-face post-meeting socialising. It remains to be seen whether this format will help these professional and social exchanges to survive.

This port-of-call is the market-place where all the various CME brands are displayed on the quayside. There are now so many that choice is difficult, but it does offer opportunities for new and rewarding CME.

REFERENCES

1. Gagnon MP, Ngangue P, Payne-Gagnon J, Desmartis M. m-Health adoption by healthcare professionals: a systematic review. *Journal of the American Medical Informatics Association* 2016;23(1):212–220. doi:10.1093/jamia/ocv052
2. UpToDate. https://www.uptodate.com/home
3. Edocate. https://edocate.com
4. ONCOassist. https://oncoassist.com
5. Giurgiu L. Microlearning an evolving elearning trend. *Science Bulletin* 2017;22(1):18–23.
6. Buchem I, Hamelmann H. Microlearning: a strategy for ongoing professional development. *eLearning Papers* 2010;21(7):1–15.
7. Bannister J, Neve M, Kolanko C. Increased educational reach through a micro-learning approach: can higher participation translate to improved outcomes? *Journal of European CME* 2020;9:1–5. doi:10.1080/21614083.2020.1834761
8. Schein EH. On dialogue, culture, and organizational learning. *Organizational Dynamics* 1993;22(2):40–51. doi:10.1016/0090-2616(93)90052-3
9. Hoadley CM, Kilner PG. Using technology to transform communities of practice into knowledge- building communities. *ACM SIGGROUP Bulletin* 2005;25(1):31–40. doi:10.1136/bmj.h4630
10. Kane B, Luz S. Information sharing at multidisciplinary medical team meetings. *Group Decision and Negotiation* 2011;20:437–464. doi:10.1007/s10726-009-9175-9
11. Nisbet G, Dunn S, Lincoln M. Interprofessional team meetings: opportunities for informal interprofessional learning. *Journal of Interprofessional Care* 2015;29(5):426–432. doi:10.3109/13561820.2015.1016602.
12. Cervero RM, Gaines JK. The impact of CME on physician performance and patient health outcomes: an updated synthesis of systematic reviews. *Journal of Continuing Education in the Health Professions* 2015;35(2):131–138. doi:10.1002/chp.21290.
13. Stevenson RD, Moore DE. Ascent to the summit of the CME pyramid. *JAMA* 2018;319(6):543–544.
14. Moore DE, Green JS, Gallis HA. Achieving the desired results and improved outcomes: integrating planning and assessment throughout learning activities. *Journal of Continuing Education in the Health Professions* 2009;29(1):1–15.
15. Porter CM. Revisiting precede–proceed: a leading model for ecological and ethical health promotion. *Health Education Journal* 2016;75(6):753–764. doi:10.1177/0017896915619645
16. Merrill MD. First principles of instruction. *ETR&D* 2002;50:43–59. doi:10.1007/BF02505024
17. Formative assessment. https://www.oecd.org/site/educeri21st/40600533.pdf
18. Lucero KS, Chen P. What do reinforcement and confidence have to do with it? a systematic pathway analysis of knowledge, competence, confidence, and intention to change. *Journal of European CME* 2020;9:1. doi:10.1080/21614083.2020.1834759

19. Accreditation Council for Continuing Medical Education (ACCME®) 2013 Annual Report Executive Summary. https://www.accme.org/sites/default/files/2019-07/630_20140715_2013_Annual_Report.pdf

20. Accreditation Council for Continuing Medical Education (ACCME®) 2019 Report. https://www.accme.org/sites/default/files/2020-07/872_2020%20 07%2028_2019_Data_Report.pdf

21. McCoy L, Lewis JH, Dalton D. Gamification and multimedia for medical education: a landscape review. *The Journal of the American Osteopathic Association* 2016;116:22–34. doi:10.7556/jaoa.2016.003

22. Lucero KS, Spyropoulos J, Blevins D, Warters M, Norton A, Cohen J. Virtual patient simulation in continuing education: improving the use of guideline-directed care in venous thromboembolism treatment. *Journal of European CME* 2020;9:1. doi:10.1080/21614083.2020.1836865

23. Cook DA, Levinson AJ, Garside S, Dupras DM, Erwin PJ, Montori VM. Internet-based learning in the health professions: a meta-analysis. *JAMA* 2008;300(10):1181–1196. doi:10.1001/jama.300.10.1181

24. Swadron SP, Herbert M. How do I effectively use electronic continuing medical education? *CJEM* 2011 Jan;13(1):40–43. doi:10.2310/8000.2011.100377

25. Cook DA, Hatala R, Brydges R, Zendejas B, Szostek JH, Wang AT, Erwin PJ, Hamstra SJ. Technology-enhanced simulation for health professions education: a systematic review and meta-analysis. *JAMA* 2011;306(9):978–988. doi:10.1001/jama.2011.1234.

26. Cook DA, Brydges R, Zendejas B, Hamstra SJ, Hatala R. Mastery learning for health professionals using technology-enhanced simulation: a systematic review and meta-analysis. *Academic Medicine* 2013;88(8):1178–1186. doi:10.1097/ACM.0b013e31829a365d.

27. Casebeer L, Brown J, Roepke N, Grimes C, Henson B, Palmore R, Granstaff US, Salinas GD. Evidence-based choices of physicians: a comparative analysis of physicians participating in Internet CME and non-participants. *BMC Medical Education* 2010;10:42. doi:10.1186/1472-6920-10-42

28. Health professions education: a bridge to quality. *National Academies Press* Washington DC. 2003. https://www.ncbi.nlm.nih.gov/books/NBK221525/?report=reader

29. Regnier K, Chappell K, Travlos DV. The role and rise of interprofessional continuing education. *Journal of Medical Regulation* 2019;105(3):6–13. doi:10.30770/2572-1852-105.3.6

30. Reeves S, Fletcher S, Barr H, Birch I, Boet S, Davies N, McFadyen A, Rivera J, Kitto S. A BEME systematic review of the effects of interprofessional education: BEME Guide No. 39. *Medical Teacher* 2016;38(7):656–668. doi:10.3109/0142159X.2016.1173663

Outcome Assessment 7

WORKPLACE INFORMAL CME

There is a lack of outcome data for informal workplace CME, but recent studies published in a Special Collection in the *Journal of European CME* are encouraging. UpToDate surveyed participants in COVID searches between January and August 2020 and found that over 94% reported that they modified their management strategies as a result of using UpToDate, and 97% reported that use of UpToDate led to improvement in care. Data from reflections necessary for awards of credits indicated reinforcement of learners' clinical management strategies in over 60% of cases with modification of their strategies in almost 30% of cases [1]. In addition to general medical databases like UpToDate, there are also highly specialised mobile apps such as the oncology decision-support tool, ONCOassist. A recent study claimed that it resulted in higher quality of care and patient safety by facilitating critical decisions at the point-of-care [2].

MDTMs have become an important medium for CME but are barely recognised as such. Little thought is given to maximise their educational potential. Hospital CME departments where they exist should welcome the opportunity to examine the educational component of MDTMs and experiment with different meeting formats to maximise the effect. This subject offers the potential for important and exciting research and just now seems to be a blank slate.

Although there are few studies on outcomes from informal CME, its very immediacy makes its effectiveness self-evident. It is like an orphan child, owned by no one, wandering about, helping physicians and patients but unrecognised for what it is. The CME community should become aware of the newcomer in its midst, take ownership of it and help it to become even more effective.

DOI: 10.1201/9781003270287-7

EXTERNAL FORMAL CME

As mentioned before, the CME community has made enormous efforts to show that formal CME planned and delivered according to defined criteria does result in positive outcomes in knowledge, performance and patient health. It is therefore argued that any future CME, similarly prepared, can be assumed to result in a satisfactory outcome. That being so, it should not be necessary for CME programmes to include outcome assessment. An analogy would be the testing and subsequent use of vaccines. During trials of a new vaccine, a satisfactory antibody response must be shown before the vaccine can be administered to the population. But it is not considered necessary to measure the antibody level in everyone who later receives the vaccine.

The counterargument runs that it is not as easy to prepare and deliver CME as it is simply to inject a vaccine. The CME gap analysis (needs assessment) may have been wrongly interpreted, a teachable moment may not have been created, the type of education may have been inappropriate or there may have been no reinforcement. Therefore, some form of outcome assessment is always necessary. However, it is admitted that conclusive proof that the PPG has been repaired in all cases is unrealistic. To do this for formal CME would need detailed pre- and post-tests and subsequent scrutiny of patient health records. This would be labour-intensive and costly – a Rolls-Royce model.

It is often reasonable to settle for the Ford or VW option. Modern pre- and post-testing using multiple choice questions (MCQs) may not measure performance but does give an indication of competence [3]. MCQs are considered to have good reliability and validity with objective scoring and to be feasible at reasonable cost [4]. The main problem is designing high-quality questions (items) to test clinical reasoning and problem-solving. It is important that the item stem should describe a clinical vignette or scenario rather than simply require factual recall [5]. It is difficult to devise such questions and to design answers, which are credible yet incorrect. The cost of their creation may be considerable.

CME providers must have, or must obtain, expertise in the science of psychometric analysis to find out whether a question is contributing to a fair verdict on the participant. The difficulty index (DIF I) describes the percentage of participants who correctly answer an MCQ and ranges from 0% to 100%. The lower the percentage, the harder the item and vice versa. Random guessing should result in 25% of the participants answering an item with four options correctly. Therefore, it is reasonable to have DIF I between the recommended range of 30%–70%. The discrimination index of an item (DI) describes the relationship between getting an MCQ correct and the overall score. It ranges between −1.00 and +1.00, with values greater than +0.30 indicating that the item is performing reasonably well. An item with a high DI value indicates that participants who had high tests scores got the correct item answer while participants who had low test scores got the wrong item answer [6].

The four or five possible answers include the one correct answer and three of four incorrect answers (distractors). The distractors should be plausible. A non-functional distractor (NFD) in an item is an option selected by fewer than 5% of participants. Distractor efficiency (DE) ranges from 0% to 100% and indicates the number of NFDs in an item – if there are none, the DE is 100%. An ideal item will have a DIF I between 30% and 70%, a DI of greater than 0.4 and a DE of 100% [6].

MCQs not only allow a participant's ability to be assessed they also of themselves contribute to learning by formative assessment in test-enhanced learning. Canadian paediatricians attending a national CPD conference experienced enhanced learning with a moderate effect size when they took part in pre- and post-MCQ testing. Feedback from post-testing helps participants to recognise areas of poor understanding [7].

A good MCQ will give a measure of competence in addition to knowledge, but the pathway from learning how to do something to actually doing it is not simple. It is influenced by many agencies, both personal and environmental. The interplay of these various factors is the essence of Social Cognitive Theory [8]. One of the most important intermediates between competence and performance is confidence, known as self-efficacy to psychologists and educationalists. Clever children lacking self-confidence do less well at mathematics than less clever children who are confident. A recent CME study found that commitment to change (CTC) was related to confidence which itself was increased by feedback in formative assessment [9]. Post-CME reflection can be considered as part of formative assessment and has been said to predispose to CTC [10] which itself has been shown to predict actual change [11]. These various findings allow CME providers to look for surrogates for performance change. It is easier to measure competence and confidence by pre- and post-testing and record reflections on CTC than trying to demonstrate a change in physician performance.

EFFECT SIZE

In recent years, the CME community has made much of the evidence showing that CME does work, reviewed by Cervero and Gaines [12]. Critics have responded by asking "To what extent does it work?"

Cervero and Gaines analysed five systemic reviews to reach their conclusion, but three of them contained no quantitative measurement [13–15]. Indeed one of them stated that "the heterogeneous nature of the studies precludes a quantitative summary of the effectiveness of CME" [11]. One study used the median adjusted risk difference to conclude that the effect on clinical practice was small to moderate with a smaller effect on patient outcomes [16]. The fifth study was the only meta-analysis and effect size was expressed as Pearson's correlation coefficient (r) with 95% confidence intervals. It similarly concluded that the effect size on physician knowledge was medium, but the effect on physician performance and patient outcome was small [17].

This illustrates that not all CME researchers have an intimate relationship with the mysterious world of statistics, but they should try to develop one. Many CME interventions assess outcome by comparison of pre- and post-test answers either expressed by a Likert scale or the results of an MCQ. The difference between the pre- and post-test means can be assumed to be statistically significant when the P-value is equal to or less than 0.05, but that gives no indication of the magnitude of the effect. If the sample size is sufficiently large, even a trivial effect size may appear to be significant, statistically but not clinically [18]. Therefore, the answer to the question about the extent of the effect of CME needs more than measurement of statistical probability.

The effect of sample size can be eliminated by using the standardised mean difference or Cohen's d, calculated by dividing the difference in the two group means (post-test mean minus pre-test mean) by their average "pooled" standard deviation (SD). This is the most suitable index to use with continuous variables. Cohen's d is expressed in SD units where a result of 0.2 indicates a small effect, 0.5 a medium effect and 0.8 a large effect. It allows comparison between the effect sizes of different CME activities and can be calculated online [19]. However, its limitation is that it can only easily be used for continuous (interval) data. Dealing with categorical variables is more complicated and requires initial calculation of Cramer's V and then conversion to Cohen's d [20].

Other indices for between-group effect size include odds ratio (OR), relative risk (RR) and risk difference (RD). In addition, there is an alternative approach to effect size using measures of association such as Pearson's correlation coefficient (Pearson's r) which can be converted to Cohen's d and vice versa [21]. Calculation of Pearson's r is carried out online [22], and a value of 0.04 indicates a small effect, 0.09 a medium effect and 0.25 a large effect.

LIMITATIONS OF SELF-REPORTED PRE- AND POST-TEST COMPARISON

When people self-report, they have a tendency to over-rate their knowledge, skills and performance in a pre-test but are more accurate in the post-test [23]. It may also be difficult to exclude a coincidental, external influence on participants in an educational intervention. Such an influence could amplify or diminish the effect of the intervention. Third, *regression to the mean* is a statistical phenomenon that can make natural variation in repeated data look like real change. It happens when unusually large or small measurements are followed by measurements that are closer to the mean [24]. When CME providers attempt to assess the outcome of their interventions, they must be aware of these factors which could affect their assessment, but they are an unavoidable evil. However, in research studies, the inclusion of a control group, which does not participate in the intervention, is necessary to allow these potentially confounding variables to be discounted.

In general, outcome assessment is increasingly evident in our competitive society. After most online transactions, the companies involved besiege us with enquiries about the service they have provided, sometimes even requesting us to complete a Likert scale. We should not find this so annoying since they are just engaging in outcome assessment in the same way as CME providers. The two situations are not entirely analogous because the award of credits to physicians may be contingent on their recording their reflections. If the physicians condemn the education as being worthless or commercially biased, would they be justified in receiving credits? This consideration may induce physicians to temper their criticism, which rather defeats the purpose of the exercise. It also questions the validity of the credit award system. Perhaps discussion among the passengers on our voyage will suggest a better currency for CME transactions.

REFERENCES

1. Damaske J, Walsh W, McKay J. CME in the time of COVID-19: educating healthcare professionals at the point-of-care and improving performance outcomes. *Journal of European CME* 2020;9:1. doi:10.1080/21614083.2020.1832798

2. Jacob C, Sanchez-Vazquez A, Ivory C. Clinicians' role in the adoption of an oncology decision support app in Europe and its implications for organizational practices: qualitative case study. *JMIR Mhealth Uhealth* 2019;7(5):e13555. https://mhealth.jmir.org/2019/5/e13555; doi:10.2196/13555

3. Tangianu F, Mazzone A, Berti F, Pinna G, Bortolotti I. Colombo F, Nozzoli C, La Regina M, Greco A, Filannino C, Silingardi M, Nardi R. Are multiple-choice questions a good tool for the assessment of clinical competence in internal medicine? *Italian Journal of Medicine* 2018;12(2):88–96. doi:10.4081/itjm.2018.980

4. Gerhard-Szep S, Güntsch A, Pospiech P, Söhnel A, Scheutzel P, Wassmann T, Zahn T. Assessment formats in dental medicine: an overview. *GMS Journal for Medical Education* 2016;33(4):Doc65. doi:10.3205/zma001064.

5. Shumway JM, Harden RM. Association for medical education in E. AMEE Guide No. 25: the assessment of learning outcomes for the competent and reflective physician. *Medical Teacher* 2003;25:569–584. doi:10.1080/0142159032000151907.

6. Sahoo DP, Singh R. Item and distracter analysis of multiple choice questions (MCQs) from a preliminary examination of undergraduate medical students. *International Journal of Research in Medical Sciences* 2017;5(12):5351–5355.

7. Feldman M, Fernando O, Wan M, Martimianakis MA, Kulasegaram K. Testing test-enhanced continuing medical education: a randomized controlled trial. *Academic Medicine* 2018;93:S30–S36. doi:10.1097/ACM.0000000000002377

8. Bandura A. Perceived self-efficacy in cognitive development and functioning. *Educational Psychologist* 1993;28(2): 117–148.

9. Lucero KS, Chen P. What do reinforcement and confidence have to do with it? A systematic pathway analysis of knowledge, competence, confidence, and intention to change. *Journal of European CME* 2020;9:1. doi:10.1080/21614083.2020.1834759

10. Ratelle JT, Wittich CM, Yu RC, Newman JS, Jenkins SM, Beckman TJ. Relationships Between Reflection and Behavior Change in CME. *Journal of Continuing Education in the Health Professions* 2017;37(3):161–167. doi:10.1097/CEH.0000000000000162.

11. Wakefield J, Herbert CP, Maclure M, Dormuth C, Wright JM, Legare J, Brett-MacLean P, Premi J. Commitment to change statements can predict actual change in practice. *Journal of Continuing Education in the Health Professions* 2003;23:81–92. doi:10.1002/chp.1340230205

12. Cervero RM, Gaines JK. The impact of CME on physician performance and patient health outcomes: an updated synthesis of systematic reviews. *Journal of Continuing Education in the Health Professions* 2015;35(2):131–8. doi:10.1002/chp.21290.

13. Davis D, Galbraith R; American College of Chest Physicians Health and Science Policy Committee. Continuing medical education effect on practice performance: effectiveness of continuing medical education: American College of Chest Physicians Evidence-Based Educational Guidelines. *Chest.* 2009;135(3 Suppl):42S–48S. doi:10.1378/chest.08-2517.

14. Mazmanian PE, Davis DA, Galbraith R. American College of Chest Physicians Health and Science Policy Committee. Continuing medical education effect on clinical outcomes: effectiveness of continuing medical education: American College of Chest Physicians Evidence-Based Educational Guidelines. *Chest* 2009;135(3 Suppl):49S–55S. doi:10.1378/chest.08-2518. PMID: 19265076.

15. Marinopoulos SS, Dorman T, Ratanawongsa N, Wilson LM, Ashar BH, Magaziner JL, Miller RG, Thomas PA, Prokopowicz GP, Qayyum R, Bass EB. Effectiveness of continuing medical education. *Evidence Report/Technology Assessment* 2007;149:1–69.

16. Forsetlund L, Bjørndal A, Rashidian A, Jamtvedt G, O'Brien MA, Wolf F, Davis D, Odgaard-Jensen J, Oxman AD. Continuing education meetings and workshops: effects on professional practice and health care outcomes. *Cochrane Database of Systematic Reviews* 2009;15(2):CD003030. doi:10.1002/14651858. CD003030.pub2.

17. Mansouri M, Lockyer J. A meta-analysis of continuing medical education effectiveness. *Journal of Continuing Education in the Health Professions* 2007;27(1):6–15. doi:10.1002/chp.88.

18. Kim HY. Statistical notes for clinical researchers: effect size. *Restorative Dentistry and Endodontics* 2015;40(4):328–331. doi:10.5395/rde.2015.40.4.328

19. Cohen's d calculation. https://lbecker.uccs.edu

20. Categorical family: effect sizes for associations among categorical variables. https://en.wikipedia.org/wiki/Effect_size#Categorical_family:_Effect_sizes_ for_associations_among_categorical_variables

21. Kim HY. Statistical notes for clinical researchers: risk difference, risk ratio, and odds ratio. *Restorative Dentistry and Endodontics* 2017;42(1):72–76. doi:10.5395/rde.2017.42.1.72

22. Pearson Correlation Coefficient Calculator. Social Science Statistics. https:// www.socscistatistics.com/tests/pearson/default2.aspx

23. My environmental education evaluation resource assistant. https://meera.snre. umich.edu/types-evaluation-designs

24. Barnett AG, van der Pols JC, Dobson AJ. Regression to the mean: what it is and how to deal with it. *International Journal of Epidemiology* 2005;34(1):215–220.

Accreditation 8

When the voyage reaches the Grand Harbour of Accreditation, a naive passenger who is a stranger in this new place would be puzzled. Why must continuing education for the healthcare professions be accredited when it is not necessary for engineers, scientists or lawyers? If accreditation is so important, why are there two entirely different ways of doing it? Why does the CME community not compare both methods and adopt the one that is better? Why do many accreditors only consider formal CME and ignore informal, workplace CME, which may be more relevant to everyday clinical practice? The answers to these questions lie in the history of accreditation.

NORTH AMERICA

During the 1960s and early 1970s, some of the more populous states in the US, enacted legislation requiring physicians to undertake a mandatory amount of CME for continued licensure. Initially, the individual states tried to regulate this process themselves, but it was felt that there was a need for a single national system to accredit CME. The Liaison Committee on Continuing Medical Education was formed in the 1970s, funded by the American Medical Association, and in 1981, its name was changed to the Accreditation Council for Continuing Medical Education (ACCME). Its main function was to accredit organisations and institutions that provide CME. To do this, it recruited volunteers who were trained to assess the activities of education providers and decide whether they met the requirements of ACCME's guidelines. This was *provider accreditation* in contrast to *activity accreditation* where individual CME interventions are submitted for prospective accreditation. At that time, the ACCME favoured a planning model based on a curriculum rather than directed by practice needs.

In 1983, the ACCME decided to limit its activities to national providers and to devolve accreditation of local providers to their state and territorial medical societies. To do this, the ACCME first accredited the state medical societies who were then empowered to accredit CME providers whose activities were carried out only within the state. In other words, the US created a two-tier system with local and national levels.

At that time, much of CME in the US was being subsidised by the pharmaceutical industry amid concerns about conflict of interests. In 1987, the ACCME issued guidelines for commercial support of CME. In 1992, more detailed standards for commercial support were adopted, which aimed at removing commercial bias designed to favour the financial interests of the company supporting the CME.

In the mid-1990s, under the new leadership of Murray Kopelow and responding to the growing body of research showing that CME could positively influence physicians' performance, the ACCME moved its position from support of curriculum-based CME to learner-centred CME. It emphasised the importance of needs assessment related to practice gaps and encouraged providers to think beyond knowledge gain and to consider clinical performance and improvement in patient health. In addition, providers were enjoined to include assessment of the success or otherwise of their activities.

However, trouble was brewing. In 2005, because of concerns about the rising costs of Medicare, Senators Grassley and Baucus of the Senate Committee on Finance wrote to the major pharmaceutical firms in the US to find out whether they were funding biased CME to promote sales of their drugs and were encouraging physicians to prescribe off-label drugs. The companies were asked to respond to 12 questions about their current practice. Almost two years later, the Senators reported that although the companies claimed to comply with the ACCME regulations, opportunities for abuse still existed [1].

At the same time, in correspondence with Kopelow, the Senators stated that the ACCME relied too much on information supplied by the providers and did not themselves examine their educational material. In addition, the ACCME did not collect data on whether providers produce activities that favour either on-label or off-label products marketed by the drug companies that fund the activities. Another criticism was that the ACCME's reaction to non-compliance with its regulations was very slow and it could take up to 9 years for a provider to lose its accreditation [1,2]. It is no coincidence that the Sunshine Act was first introduced in 2007 by Senator Grassley. It was enacted along with the 2010 Patient Protection and Affordable Care Act. The Act requires manufacturers of drugs and devices to collect and track all financial relationships with physicians and teaching hospitals and to report these data to the Centers for Medicare and Medicaid Services [3].

Following the Senate Committee report, providers were required to be more scrupulous about the content of their educational material and ACCME reviewed content when complaints were lodged about possible bias. Since then, there has been a steady decline in the numbers of activities with commercial support. The ACCME annual report from 2019 stated that "the majority of CME activities (92%) did not receive commercial support, accounting for 88% of physician interactions, and 86% of other learner interactions. Eight percent of CME activities did receive commercial support, accounting for 12% of physician interactions and 14% of other learner interactions". This of course suggests that activities with commercial support were relatively more popular with learners than those without such support. The total number of CME activities in 2019 was 188,992 delivered by 1,724 providers [4].

The American Academy of Family Physicians (AAFP) has followed a different path from hospital specialists. It does not accredit providers but rather accredits individual CME activities. On average, the AAFP Credit System reviews and awards credits for about 1,300 CME provider customers, whose activities exceed 18,000 per year [5].

The US process for CME accreditation is mirrored by its northern neighbour. Canada's Royal College, like the ACCME, accredits providers of CME designed for hospital physicians and the College of Family Physicians accredits activities like the AAFP.

EUROPE

At some point in the late 20th century, European countries became aware that CME accreditation was being carried out in North America. There was a feeling that they should not be left behind, but Europe can be less than whole-hearted when it follows an American initiative. Provider accreditation, as practised by the ACCME and the Royal College in Canada, had required major financial investment to establish organisations in Chicago and Ottawa. Individual European countries balked at such expenditure and opted for what appeared to be the cheaper choice of activity accreditation. This may have been a false economy.

In Europe, each country is responsible for accrediting the ever-increasing number of its own CME activities, but to deal with CME designed for European or international learners, the European Accreditation Council for CME (EACCME) was established in 1999. The EACCME forwards CME submissions to the relevant Specialist Section of the European Union of Medical Specialists (UEMS) which is the parent organisation of the EACCME. The submission is also sent to the National Accreditation Authority (NAA) of the country which is hosting the educational activity. Both of these organisations have to approve the submission before it is accredited. However, the

EACCME deals with only the small fraction of European activities designed for international learners – 1759 activities in 2019 [6]. These represent a tiny minority of the total. For example, in part of one of the German Länder, Westphalia-Lippe, there were 33,855 submissions for CME activities in 2019 and of these only 34 were rejected. In other words, 99.9% of submissions were accredited [7]. Most European NAAs and the EACCME do not publish their rejection rates, but they are likely to be similar to the German data. It is not surprising that with so many submissions, the vast majority would be approved, but it is reasonable to ask if there is any point in persisting with an examination with a pass rate of that order. In contrast, in the US, a provider can be examined by the ACCME every 4 of 6 years and, if found to be satisfactory, is empowered to provide CME unhindered until its next review.

Kopelow and Campbell compared the two systems [8] and claimed that provider accreditation was associated with an *economy of scale*. They illustrated this with data from 2008 to 2012 during which the EACCME approved 6500 activities. During a similar time frame (2008 to 2011), the ACCME made more than 700 accreditation decisions and its accredited providers reported 365,718 CME activities. This was more than a 500:1 ratio of activities to accreditation decisions by the ACCME system while the EACCME maintained a 1:1 ratio. Of course, each ACCME decision was reached after an intensive and expensive review of the provider's previous performance, whereas an EACCME decision just required prospective scrutiny of a single, proposed educational activity.

The Europeans counter this by referring back to 2007 when the ACCME was held responsible for not examining educational material sponsored by the drug industry and which unfairly promoted their sales. They also remind the Americans of the inordinate length of time it takes for a non-compliant provider to lose its accreditation. The ACCME would say that these loopholes in their review process have now been fixed.

Kopelow and Campbell also adduce evidence that suggests that accepting and complying with their accreditation criteria promote a "community of practice" among providers which encourages their development and offers membership of an academy for the scholarly pursuit of continuing education [8]. No one has ever suggested that the European system encourages a community of practice and indeed it is not popular with the providers, particularly European specialist societies, who find the need for dual accreditation time-consuming and expensive.

There is an important difference in the type of people who must be recruited to operate the two accreditation systems. Provider accreditation requires that the activities of a provider be critically examined in terms of PPG discovery and analysis (needs assessment), CME design, predisposition, enabling and reinforcement, followed by outcome assessment. These are generic activities and are not specialty-specific. For example, a gastroenterologist could assess the quality of a provider whose activities were exclusively aimed at cardiologists. On the other hand, in activity accreditation, reliable review of a proposed CME intervention in cardiology would have to be done by a cardiologist.

The European Union (EU) and European Economic Area (EEA) recognise 55 clinical specialties [9]. There are over 30 countries in the EU and the EAA. Ideally, each country should have specialty reviewers for each specialty, although in practice, this does not happen because the number would be prohibitively high. Nevertheless, a great many physicians are involved in national CME accreditation in Europe. The EACCME has 43 specialist sections [10], each with a CME/CPD subcommittee. As noted above, they reviewed 1759 submissions in 2019 delivered at the European or international level [6]. The ACCME in the US has approximately 165 volunteers who were responsible for 96,663 activities in 2019 delivered at the national level [11]. These recent data further support Kopelow and Campbell's claim of an *economy of scale* made almost a decade earlier [8].

The increasing significance of informal CME presents more problems for activity accreditors. Point-of-care CME is unpremeditated micro-learning and it is difficult to see how every individual episode could be accredited as an educational activity. MDTMs are planned workplace events, but they are so numerous and disparate that activity accreditation would be impractical. Therefore, although practising physicians do not dispute the importance of informal workplace CME, learners under the jurisdiction of activity accreditors cannot easily be credited for their informal CME. Indeed, it is questionable whether activity accreditors even recognise this as a problem. In the paper on CPD from the Federation of the Royal Colleges of Physicians of the UK, updated in 2020, there is no mention of point-of-care CME or MDTMs [12].

On the other hand, provider accreditors have no such difficulties. Accredited providers such as UpToDate automatically award credits on a time basis for all registered users who can access their credit history at any time. Accredited hospital CME departments can award learners with credits for attending MDTMs or Patient Care Conferences. Not only do such learners get well-deserved credits but ideally the CME department would have optimised the educational value of the meetings as should have been required of it by the accreditor during the submission process. That said, there is not much indication that the accreditation establishment in general recognises the increasing importance of workplace CME. In the recently presented *Standards for Substantive Equivalency* from the *International Academy for CPD Accreditation*, only one sentence in Domain 5 refers to "workplace learning", and as with the Federation above, there is no allusion to point-of-care CME or MDTMs [13].

The nomenclature can be confusing for newcomers to the world of CME. Activities or providers are *accredited*, and the provider awards *credits* to the learners after they have taken part in the education. The usual criterion for the number of credits awarded is one hour – one credit. Increasingly, the acquisition of credits is becoming mandatory, although some countries still operate a voluntary system. Individual countries all decide the minimum number of credits their physicians must earn either on an annual of 5-yearly basis and they also stipulate the proportion of credits to be obtained from the different forms of CME – clinical, non-clinical, formal external, informal internal and eLearning.

To those of us who care about CME, the award of CME credits based on an hourly rate is demeaning. By complying with this, we let the currency of our discipline be degraded by an unworthy criterion. It is not unreasonable for physicians to expect that the commitment they make to CME will be recognised and appreciated, but preferably on the basis of the effort they have expended and the benefit they have received. The CME community will never be accorded the respect it deserves until it finds a better way to measure a physician's engagement with CME.

It is possible to envisage a European system analogous to the US, where a European accreditation agency adopted provider accreditation and invited all the NAAs to apply for provider accreditation in the same way that the ACCME accredits the state medical societies. Then the accredited NAAs would accredit their own national providers and the European agency would accredit the international or European providers. The present authorities would not agree to a scheme such as this. In his annual report in 2016, the Secretary-General of the UEMS, said that "While we continue to categorically oppose provider accreditation ...." [14]. However, the specialist societies, who are the main European providers, may take a different view and, if so, could use their influence and considerable financial resources to encourage a European reappraisal of its present system.

ACCREDITATION STANDARDS – PHARMACEUTICAL INDUSTRY

The pharmaceutical industry has always provided CME for physicians to inform them of its products. The current consensus holds that such CME should not be accredited. A drug company may however support accredited CME by publishing a Request for Proposal for an educational activity related to a disease state for which it produces drug treatment. The company would pay the CME provider whose proposal was accepted but would have to maintain an arm's length relationship with the provider and must not influence the selection of faculty, educational design or outcome assessment. The standards to which the industry must adhere are described by the ACCME [15] and by the European Federation of Pharmaceutical Industries and Associations (EFPIA) [16]. Some companies in the drug industry do not accept that their present exclusion from accredited CME is justified. In the most frequently viewed paper in the lifetime of the *Journal of European CME*, seven authors from various companies argue for *collaborative partnerships* in the provision of accredited CME [17]. The accreditation establishment in both the US [18] and in Europe [19] was quick to respond with unequivocal rebuttals.

Having absorbed the foregoing, the naive passenger in the first paragraph will now know that accreditation is considered necessary first because CME is becoming increasingly important for Maintenance of Certification and revalidation, to a much greater degree than continuing education in other professions. Second, drug firms cannot always be trusted to honestly represent the proper use of their drugs and third, physicians cannot always be trusted to resist the improper representations of drug firms. The passenger will also know that provider accreditation may be more user-friendly and practical than activity accreditation, but will not understand why proponents of the latter are so adamant in their refusal to consider that a change might be sensible. In addition, the passenger will have understood that accreditation of informal CME presents no problem for provider accreditation but that activity accreditation is ill-suited to this type of CME, which is becoming increasingly important.

Lastly, the previously naive passenger might still wonder why the disciples of accreditation have seen no need to prove to a sceptical world that the degree of improvement in patient health attributed to accreditation, justifies the time and money invested in it. At present, it is not cheap to anchor in the Grand Harbour of Accreditation.

REFERENCES

1. Responses from pharmaceutical drug and device makers to Grassley request for disclosure of support for continuing medical education. *United States Senate Committee on Finance.* 2008 https://www.finance.senate.gov/ranking-members-news/responses-from-pharmaceutical-drug-and-device-makers-to-grassley-request-for-disclosure-of-support-for-continuing-medical-education
2. Commercial Sponsorship of Continuing Medical Education. *Testimony before the Senate Special Committee on Aging* 2009. https://www.oig.hhs.gov/testimony/docs/2009/07292009_oig_testimony.pdf

3. Everything you need to know about the Sunshine Act. *BMJ* 2013;347:f4704. doi:10.1136/bmj.f4704

4. Accreditation Council for Continuing Medical Education. 2020. ACCME Data Report: Steady Growth in Accredited Continuing Medical Education – 2019. www.accme.org/2019datareport. https://www.accme.org/sites/default/files/2020-07/872_2020%2007%2028_2019_Data_Report.pdf

5. AAFP Credit System 2021. https://www.aafp.org/cme/credit-system.html

6. UEMS Secretary-general report 2020. https://www.uems.eu/__data/assets/pdf_file/0005/123494/SG-report-OCT2020.pdf

7. Bericht des Vorstandes der Ärztekammer Westfalen-Lippe 2019; 54. https://www.aekwl.de/fileadmin/user_upload/aekwl/aerztekammer/dokumente/Vorstandsbericht_2019_fin.pdf

8. Kopelow M, Campbell C. The benefits of accrediting institutions and organisations as providers of continuing professional education. *Journal of European CME* 2013;2:10–14. doi:10.3109/21614083.2013.779580

9. EUR-Lex, Access to European Union Law 2020. https://eur-lex.europa.eu/legal-content/EN/LSU/?uri=CELEX:32005L0036

10. UEMS Medical Specialities 2013. https://www.uems.eu/about-us/medical-specialties

11. ACCME Data Report supplement 2019. https://www.accme.org/sites/default/files/2020-07/873_20200728_2019_Supplement_Report.pdf

12. Federation of the Royal Colleges of Physicians of the United Kingdom 2020. https://9def6877-09ab-4e8b-ae26-a9364135cfc2.filesusr.com/ugd/8f8bf8_a59500a206ac4c65b81ab2466165f068.pdf

13. International Academy for CPD Accreditation, Standards for Substantive Equivalency 2020. https://academy4cpdaccreditation.files.wordpress.com/2020/10/final_iacpda_standards_for_substantive_equivalency_10072020.pdf

14. UEMS Council Meeting, Report of the Secretary General 2016. https://www.uems.eu/__data/assets/pdf_file/0013/40306/UEMS-2016.01-Secretary-General-Report-October-2016.pdf

15. ACCME Accreditation Requirements 2020. https://www.accme.org/sites/default/files/2020-12/626_20201210_Accreditation_Requirements.pdf

16. EFPIA Code On The Promotion of Prescription-Only Medicines To, And Interactions With, Healthcare Professionals 2014. https://www.efpia.eu/media/24302/3a_efpia-hcp-code-2014.pdf

17. Allen T, Donde N, Hofstädter-Thalmann E, Keijser S, Moy V, Jean-Jacques Murama J-J, Kellner T. Framework for industry engagement and quality principles for industry-provided medical education in Europe. *Journal of European CME* 2017;6:1, 1348876. doi: 10.1080/21614083.2017.1348876

18. McMahon GT. Independence from industry cannot be compromised, *Journal of European CME*. 2017;6:1, 1393296. doi: 10.1080/21614083.2017.1393296

19. Griebenow R. Industry 1/m from sponsor to provider? *Journal of European CME* 2017;6:1, 1395672. doi: 10.1080/21614083.2017.1395672

Continuing Professional Development and Fitness to Practise

9

All people *develop* for good or ill as they try to come to terms with the vicissitudes of life. Professional people are no more or less liable to *develop* well or badly but are usually better organised. Leaders of professions have now assumed responsibility for supervising the CPD of their members and they have established organisations for that purpose. In many cases, such organisations arrange regular appraisal sessions with members.

First, they try to detect members who have gone *rogue* so that they can protect the public from their malevolent activities. Second, they have a duty of care to help those members who are not coping with the demands made of them. Third, they must encourage all the other members to direct their development for the betterment of those whom they serve.

In healthcare, as mentioned in the first chapter, CPD is quite different from CME. The concept of CPD arose because of the lecture room connotation of traditional didactic CME, which was also seen as too narrow to encompass all the aspects of physicians' behaviour [1,2]. Discussion on this topic took place in the 1990s when the CME community in the US and Canada was busily engaged in trying to discover why CME was not effective. These studies were successful and did provide the answer to the question of how to plan and deliver effective CME [3]. If only the malcontents had been more patient and waited for a few more years, they might not have needed to invent a new name for a supposedly failing system.

Nevertheless, it is useful to assess physicians' behaviour not just in terms of their clinical performance but also to take into account other factors that

DOI: 10.1201/9781003270287-9

contribute to their professional development. CPD cannot be provided by an external agency like CME, but rather must be planned and carried out by physicians themselves in response to circumstances that may be inimical not only to optimal clinical performance but also to their well-being and career prospects.

CME is of course intimately involved in the learner's CPD. No physician can hope to perform adequately without up-to-date knowledge and skills. Therefore, the professional body charged with monitoring CPD must first and foremost examine the learners' CME portfolios. This can be done at the most basic and unimaginative level by checking that the learners have collected the requisite minimum number of CME credits, regardless of any effect on clinical competence or performance. A more discriminating and less mechanistic alternative is to use an annual appraisal to make a qualitative rather than a quantitative assessment of the previous year's CME activities. This is more demanding than credit number crunching, but may do more to enhance the standing of CME in the eyes of the profession.

In addition to their CME history, physicians must also adduce evidence from recent activities to reassure the peer-appraiser that CPD has been effectively achieved. This will include details of critical incidents, interprofessional relationships and tensions, timely patient access to care and response to complaints. The appraiser must be wary of the evidence. There is still doubt whether Dr Harold Shipman, who murdered more than 200 of his patients, would have been exposed by appraisal [4].

Third-party information should be available. Many countries use multisource feedback (MSF), also known as the 360-degree feedback with responses from colleagues, nurses and patients. MSF requires that questionnaires be designed to determine competence for specific behavioural tasks. A steering committee must ensure that the questions on behaviour are appropriate. The MSF is a flexible instrument and allows questions to be customised for different respondents (raters). For example, the patient instrument would focus on professionalism, interpersonal and communication skills, whereas the colleague instrument would cover medical knowledge and patient care. It must be checked for reliability and to determine whether there are sufficient numbers of raters and items on the instrument to guarantee generalisability [5]. MSF is not a suitable instrument for assessing clinical outcomes, but its strength lies in revealing interpersonal people skills, ability to communicate and engagement in team-work. Physicians can use the feedback to consider changes in practice and behaviour. They may also use self-evaluation using the colleague instrument to compare their own score with those from their colleagues. Such feedback acts as formative assessment and may result in performance change [6].

In Chapter 4, the difficulty of providing CME for physicians with poor diagnostic skills was highlighted. Physicians are sensitive about their diagnostic ability. However, it was suggested that diagnostic performance could more easily be discussed in the privacy of the CPD appraisal. Problems with diagnosis should be addressed in MSF returns and these might generate a teachable moment in the appraisee. It would be important for the appraiser to be familiar with decision-making theory, heuristic shortcuts and associated biases, metacognition, reflection and debiasing strategies.

The systems and instruments described above were created primarily to monitor physicians' CPD, but in large part they have been hijacked for a different purpose. They have come to form the basis for deciding fitness to practise. In the 1970s, time-limited certification was introduced in the US and, since 2000, Maintenance of Certification (MOC) programmes have been adopted with a 10-yearly, four-part recertification assessment of medical knowledge, competence and communication skills. This system is not mandatory and includes an examination. Canada's present system was launched in 2011 by the Royal College of Physicians and Surgeons of Canada with a revised MOC programme framework, credit system and ePortfolio. The UK revalidation system began in 2012 with annual appraisals requiring exhaustive documentation of activities. There is a more detailed appraisal every 5 years (including results from MSF) when decisions on revalidation are made. Comparable systems have been established worldwide. The cost has of course been enormous, both in time and money. It is too soon to know what will be the return on this investment. A recent survey of Responsible Officers in the UK revalidation system suggested that "one size fits all" was not the best model and that it should be more responsive to individual and professional contexts [7]. It was better in dealing with poor performance, but less useful for physicians who were performing well. In the US, where recertification is long-established, there is little evidence that it improves patient care [8].

The regulatory authorities should perhaps carry out a gap analysis in relation to future modifications of their revalidation and recertification systems and focus on areas known to affect performance. Foremost is age. In a systematic review of 62 studies, more than half suggested that physician performance declined over time for all outcomes measured [9]. In one of the studies, mortality for hospitalised patients with acute myocardial infarction increased for every year since the treating physician had graduated from medical school [10]. The General Medical Council in the UK stated that physicians who attracted more than two complaints between 2007 and 2012 were seven times more likely to receive a further complaint in 2013.

These data should prompt a reappraisal of the organisation of physicians' professional life. Is it reasonable to expect a physician at the age of 65 years to function in the same way as a physician of 25 years? Advancing age is the enemy of acute and out-of-hours medical practice. Old physicians become more easily tired and lose the hand/eye coordination they once had. Old surgeons lack the stamina for emergency operations in the middle of the night. On the other hand, many are good teachers, thrive in out-patient clinics and have managerial experience. When senior physicians request reorganisation of their duties, junior physicians often raise objections because their own workload may increase, but they should remember that they will become old themselves. It is not in anyone's interest to force on ageing physicians a work programme with which they can no longer cope. When healthcare managers and younger physicians are intransigent in reaching accommodation with senior physicians, the predictable result is that seniors take early retirement.

Cognitive impairment is closely related to age, and in a recent study of 141 clinicians aged 70 years or older, 18 clinicians (12.7%) demonstrated cognitive deficits that were likely to impair their ability to practise medicine independently [11]. A reasonable estimate of impaired physician performance appears to be 6%–12%. Age-related cognitive decline, substance use disorders and other psychiatric illness diminish physicians' insight into their level of performance as well as their ability to benefit from an educational experience [12].

The above are risk factors for physician under-performance that should be targeted in CPD appraisal. There seems to be little justification for subjecting young, healthy physicians to a huge bureaucratic exercise from which they are unlikely to derive benefit. If it is the case that appraisal with formative assessment does not improve performance in physicians already performing adequately, it is reasonable to ask if anything else would be more effective. In Chapter 2, a culture of learning is said to be promoted when healthcare institutions invest in their professionals such that they feel valued. This same strategy should similarly encourage CPD. Therefore, authorities charged with overseeing recertification and revalidation should perhaps ease back on bombarding physicians with ever more forms to be filled and instead concentrate on how to optimise the organisational culture of the hospitals and other healthcare institutions where they work.

REFERENCES

1. Atlay RD, Wentz DK. CME or CPD? *Postgraduate Medical Journal* 1996;72(suppl):S613.
2. Davis D, Barnes BE, Fox RD. *The Continuing Professional Development of Physicians: From Research to Practice*. American Medical Association Press, Chicago; 2003.
3. Cervero RM, Gaines JK. The impact of CME on physician performance and patient health outcomes: an updated synthesis of systematic reviews. *Journal of Continuing Education in the Health Professions* 2015;35(2):131–138. doi:10.1002/chp.21290. PMID: 26115113.

4. GPonline.2017.https://www.gponline.com/harold-shipman-caught-todays-nhs-says-sir-keith-pearson/article/1420762

5. Lockyer J. Multisource feedback in the assessment of physician competencies. *Journal of Continuing Education in the Health Professions* 2003;23(1):4–12. doi:10.1002/chp.1340230103

6. Narayanan, A, Farmer EA, Greco MJ. Multisource feedback as part of the Medical Board of Australia's Professional Performance Framework: Outcomes from a preliminary study. *BMC Medical Education* 2018;18:323. doi:10.1186/s12909-018-1432-7

7. Walshe K, Boyd A, Bryce M, Luscombe K, Tazzyman A, Tredinnick-Rowe J, Archer J. Implementing medical revalidation in the United Kingdom: Findings about organisational changes and impacts from a survey of responsible officers. *Journal of the Royal Society* 2017;110(1):23–30. doi:10.1177/0141076816683556

8. Maintenance of Certification. https://en.wikipedia.org/wiki/Maintenance_of_Certification

9. Choudhry NK, Fletcher RH, Soumerai SB. Systematic review: The relationship between clinical experience and the quality of health care. *Annals of Internal Medicine* 2005;142(4):260–273.

10. Norcini JJ. Current perspectives in assessment: The assessment of performance at work. *Medical Education* 2005;39:880–889.

11. Cooney L, Balcezak T. Cognitive testing of older clinicians prior to recredentialing. *JAMA* 2020;323(2):179–180. doi:10.1001/jama.2019.18665

12. Williams BW. The prevalence and special educational requirements of dyscompetent physicians. *Journal of Continuing Education in the Health Professions* 2006;26(3):173–191. doi:10.1002/chp.68

Epilogue

And so the voyage is over. At least one passenger has learnt a great deal about CME and CPD and that person is of course the author. It is his earnest hope that the passengers who responded to his invitation to accompany him on the voyage have enjoyed the learning experience. The physicians and other healthcare professionals among them will perhaps perform their clinical duties to greater effect, being able to engage more profitably in their CME.

When physicians feel uncomfortable during clinical activity, they may be more likely to recognise this as cognitive dissonance due to awareness of a new practice gap. Hopefully, they will stop and try to analyse the gap before working out how best to access the necessary CME. They should be more familiar with the opportunities for point-of-care workplace CME than previously.

Physicians should also have a deeper understanding of the difference between CME and CPD. CME will help them to deal with their patients' problems and CPD will help them to deal with their own problems. They may now see these two as their friends, instead of bureaucratic hurdles, and perhaps be more likely to discuss revalidation and recertification constructively with the regulatory authorities.

The part-time specialist society CME providers may have been pleasantly surprised to find that CME is more interesting and challenging than they previously thought. They may now be able to appreciate the skills of professional and commercial providers who would be happy to help them. European providers may have a better understanding of the regulations and accreditation processes that govern their activities. They may be emboldened to have discussions with the authorities to address concerns that they may have. European accreditors may wonder if their determined opposition to provider accreditation is justified.

The CME academics will have had the opportunity to talk to clinicians, and from this dialogue a better *modus vivendi* may develop. The European academic educationalists, not previously familiar with the world of CME, should have been impressed by the quality of the research achievements in CME. So much so, that they will hasten to recognise CME as a scholarly academic discipline, well qualified to stand alongside undergraduate medical education in European universities and medical schools.

Index

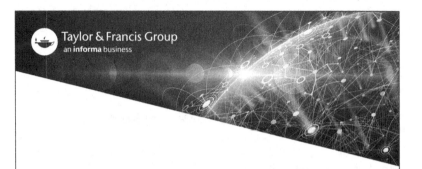